Contents

Foreword

My first son simply hated to sleep. I think he was always afraid he would miss something wonderful the moment he closed his eyes. But he was very irritable when he didn't get enough sleep! This made mothering him even more stressful than it naturally was. And, once I finally got him sleeping, it seems I blinked and he became a toddler who had opinions about everything! I blinked again and I had a little boy who was ready for the potty in order to sleep over 10 to 12 hours at night without wetting the bed.

Children change so fast, in the blink of an eye, and as a new parent, you have so many questions! Just when you figure one thing out, something else comes up. It took having my second child to teach me how children can be temperamentally different even when they grow up in the same home. This helped me become even more passionate about helping families sleep. After all, we are better, more fun, and patient parents when we get enough sleep.

For over a decade now, I have worked with thousands of families to achieve the sometimes-elusive goal of their babies and toddlers "sleeping through the night." Over the years, I've learned that one of the primary challenges in modern-day parenting is that our "village" has shrunk, if not disappeared altogether. Or, to view it another way, our "village" is now so large that there are too many voices hindering a parent's ability to learn true wisdom. This leaves many parents confused and not very confident in raising their children.

The Complete Guide to

POTTY
TRAINING

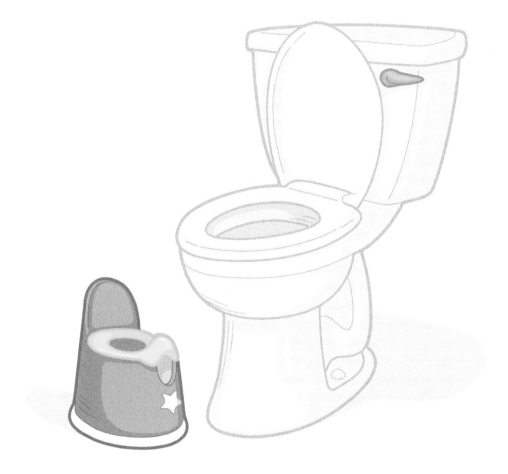

The Complete Guide to

POTTY TRAINING

The Step-by-Step Plan with Expert Solutions for Any Mess

Michelle D. Swaney

FOREWORD BY NICOLE JOHNSON
INTRODUCTION BY JENNIFER SINGER, MD

ALTHEA
PRESS

In dedication to my media naranja, Matthew.
It is a joy to be your wife.
And to our most precious gifts: Timothy, Poema, and Sierra.

I'm the mom of two similar—yet very different—boys, a parenting expert, and the Founder and Lead Sleep Consultant of The Baby Sleep Site®. I can confidently proclaim there is no one-size-fits-all solution to many parenting challenges, ranging from sleep coaching to potty training. So, when I read this book, it was like a breath of fresh air! Michelle encourages parents to personalize their child's potty training experience just like I personalize my clients' sleep coaching experience. This book will not only help you potty train your child quickly, but will also encourage and empower you as a parent. Her underlying focus on empowering your children during this process can't be overlooked.

After working with tens of thousands of parents over the years, I know that gaining confidence as a parent is the best gift you can give yourself . . . and your child. This book will answer all your pressing questions about when your child is ready for potty training as well as the most personalized way to train them. You'll learn from other parents' experiences and how to navigate your way through common troubles. Michelle even addresses how to handle things if you have a child with special needs. I can and will confidently recommend this book to my clients who need potty training help while also preserving a good night's sleep.

—Nicole Johnson

Introduction

When I first met Michelle, it was immediately evident that she cares for her children not only with compassion and love, but also with levelheadedness and sound reasoning.

As a pediatric urologist, I handle a wide variety of problems infants and children may experience, from simple management strategies for urinary tract infections to complicated urological conditions that require complex reconstructive and corrective surgeries.

A common area of my clinical practice is the management of a variety of voiding issues related to delayed toilet training and bedwetting. Parents are often referred to me wanting to know if their child is "normal" because they are having daytime or nighttime accidents. Determining whether such a child has a medical condition is one of the things that I do, and I do it often. But it's not always easy.

When toilet training goes smoothly, the experience can be enjoyable and serve as a bonding experience. When it is difficult, we need to support our children through the process.

In her approach to toilet training, Michelle is as thoughtful and grounded as she is in the care of her own children. She balances love and compassion with a practical expectation that most children can, and should, be able to toilet train just fine. She presents a reasoned and stepwise approach to the process of toilet training that can be applied to most children who are unaffected by interfering medical conditions. She has extensive experience applying her program, and she has demonstrated time and time again that it works. This book provides parents and caregivers with options that can be individualized to meet the needs of their child and family.

I especially like Tools of the Trade in chapter 3 (page 34). Here, you will find a terrific listing of materials and resources that you can tailor to your child's and family's needs in your toilet training journey. In Chapter 6: Pooping and Peeing (page 80), you will find helpful pearls of wisdom about constipation, a common issue which may interfere with the normal toilet training process or, in some cases, may actually reverse a previously trained child back to accidents. In Chapter 8: Out and About (page 102), you will find helpful recommendations about what you may need to facilitate leaving the house during the training process.

As you read this wonderful book, I encourage you to consider the unique circumstances of your child and family. Be open-minded and patient. Try not to feel overwhelmed. You will get through this. Good luck!

—Jennifer Singer, MD

Preface

I was a first-time mom to a sweet little boy—a little boy we weren't sure we were going to be able to have after the six rounds of chemotherapy I'd been through for colon cancer. But here he was, our adorable miracle, and he was already growing up. At 10 months our son was starting to walk, and I hated the thought of our little guy running around with poop in his pants. It was then I started to wonder, "What are my options for getting him to start using the toilet?" Despite being in a sleep-deprived, new-mom haze, I was able to recall a memory from earlier in my life.

I graduated college early so that I could volunteer in Nicaragua with an international medical nonprofit. I remember having lunch at a woman's house that was made of four sticks, black plastic around the sides, and a corrugated metal roof. She had multiple children, several of whom were "diaper-wearing" age, at least in the United States. It was hurricane season and it quickly started raining. Distraught, she said, "Mi un Pampers!" because her one cloth diaper was getting drenched outside. *Pampers* was the word used for any diaper there. I thought, "How does she have one diaper for two or three kids who should all be in diapers?"

That day, I followed her around, curious about how it all worked. She had potty trained her children early by learning the physical signs that they needed to go and then cueing them when it was convenient for her to have them go.

I never thought this simple memory would be the start of a now 13-year journey to become a potty training expert, but that is exactly what happened. I realized that the age-old wisdom of baby potty learning could be combined with modern-day methods. In fact, combining the two methods is the answer that so many potty training parents have been searching for.

I became a potty training expert because I was overwhelmed as a mom. I know what it's like to need more than just a digital high five. What we need is practical advice to get the job done.

As the CEO of The Potty School I have asked thousands of parents, "What's your number one potty training question?" The most frequent questions are "When should I start?" and "How should I start?" This book will give you clear answers to those two questions. I will guide you through the popular topics of pooping, nights and naps, how to leave the house, and getting out and about. You'll learn how to incorporate other family members and caregivers, and how to deal with resistance, special circumstances, and accidents. For those of you who like using extrinsic motivation, there's a progress tracker at the back as well. And we'll close with a list of valuable resources that I wish I'd had when I started this journey.

As a professional potty trainer I've consulted with many confused and frustrated parents who just needed a listening ear and some proven guidance. I've been able to save families money—families who weren't sure how they were going to afford diapers for the next year. I've been able to reduce the eco-footprint of our generation, one diaper at a time. I've helped parents foster self-mastery skills both in themselves and in their children. I've taught parents to confidently instruct their children and emphasized the opportunity to celebrate successes with their children. Those are the things that really matter. Those are the reasons I do what I do. That is what *The Complete Guide to Potty Training* is about. I want your journey to be more than just getting pee and poo in the potty; I want to help you enjoy and strengthen your relationship with your child along the way.

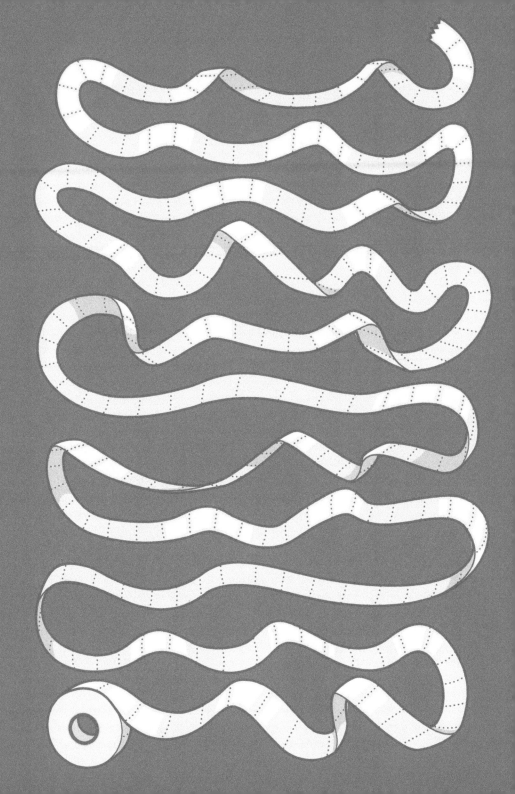

Part One

BEFORE
WE BEGIN

Setting Expectations
Is Your Child Ready?
Are You Ready?

ONE

Setting Expectations

A BIG MILESTONE

Can you believe we're even here talking about potty training your little one? When did that happen? Wasn't it just recently that you were "ooooh-ing" and "ahhhing" over the fact that diapers even came in sizes small enough for your newborn? Since then, you've probably celebrated your child's major milestones: sitting up, crawling, walking, first words, and maybe even full sentences. Or perhaps you've worried about your child being delayed in one or more of these milestones. Don't worry; as clichéd as it sounds, every child is unique and develops at their own pace. Potty training is just another major milestone in your child's development. Not only is potty training a physical development, but it's a chance for you to teach your child to be independent.

For the sake of argument, I'm going to assume that you are the child's parent or guardian and that you love them dearly. That love will greatly affect how you potty train . . . in a wonderfully transformational way!

Your child wasn't born with a diaper on. We, as the parents, put it on them. We therefore need to be the ones to teach them to use the proper receptacle. In this chapter, we are going to talk about expectations for your child and their ability to be potty trained.

This is the first time as parents that we are expecting our children to be self-aware and self-reliant, and potentially to have self-mastery of skills. We are passing the baton on to our child and saying, "You can do this and I can help!"

Potty training is a wonderful opportunity to:

- Foster your child's self-awareness
- Have a positive influence
- Teach self-mastery of skills
- Exemplify life skills
- Set the tone for how you and your child reach goals together
- Decide how you'd like to motivate your child in the long term

Let's learn more about these wonderful opportunities to teach your child skills that they can use not only during the potty training process but during the whole course of their development.

Foster Your Child's Self-Awareness

There are four stages your child will go through as far as awareness of their bodily functions goes.

Our main goal when we start potty training is to help move our child from whatever stage they are currently in, on to the next one. We want them to move to a state where they can tell us, "Mama, I need to pee pee," or "Daddy, where's the potty? I need to go." Then, if you happen to have more children, your child can also be an invaluable resource to let you know, "Sister is wiggly, I think she needs to potty." This can be a super-helpful thing if you happen to be distracted.

THE FOUR STAGES OF SELF-AWARENESS

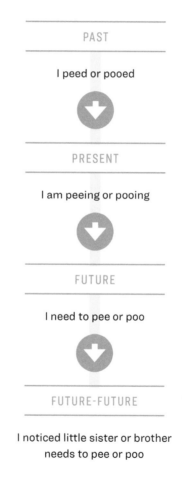

PAST

I peed or pooed

PRESENT

I am peeing or pooing

FUTURE

I need to pee or poo

FUTURE-FUTURE

I noticed little sister or brother
needs to pee or poo

I PEED OR POOED

In this stage, you will be teaching your child the difference between wet and dry so that they know if they have had an accident. You will help them notice the change and you'll teach them what to do in response.

Teaching a child not only to notice that they have soiled themselves, but that they can feel the pressure on their belly or in their lower abdomen, is very helpful. This will teach them to be aware of whether they have an upset stomach, and to feel the difference between gas and poop. This skill may mean the difference, in the middle of a long car ride, between an emergency stop on the side of the road and your child just passing gas.

If your child is developmentally delayed, these processes may involve more steps. Instead of being able to teach your child to push down and pull up their pants before and after going to the bathroom, you may need to break it down into several less complex steps. It will take more teaching, but that time will well be worth it when your delayed child is not only able to use the toilet but even initiates the process in a way that works for your family.

I AM PEEING OR POOING

This is the point where your child is actively peeing or pooing and they are realizing what's happening. Maybe they're naked and they're noticing that there's urine coming out and visually seeing it. Maybe they're pooping and feel it coming out. Whichever sense they are using to realize they are going, you can capitalize on that and use that information to encourage them to notice in the future before it happens.

I NEED TO PEE OR POO

How your kiddo conveys their need to potty depends on your child's current level of development. We are going to potty train them at the level they are currently at, not the level you want them to be when they're done. If your child is 16 months you can't expect them to say, "Where's the potty? I need to go!" That is a more reasonable expectation of a three-year-old or four-year-old child. Your child's ability to converse will determine how they will let you know they need to go; they could communicate verbally or nonverbally, using words, sign language, a bell, or tapping a parent's leg.

I NOTICED LITTLE SISTER OR BROTHER NEEDS TO PEE OR POO

This is a goal that most parents don't ever think about. They think that once their child can go to the bathroom they are set: potty training accomplished. Yes, that's true, and at that point I encourage you to do a happy dance. But as a mother of three, having my three-year-old tell me when my one-year-old needs to go to the potty is ridiculously helpful. You shouldn't be disappointed if your older child doesn't alert you if your younger child is going to the bathroom, but you can empower them to be helpful in the potty training process. Even if they can't change diapers, they can be a big help.

Have a Positive Influence

You are able to positively impact your child. When your child succeeds, you get to be the one encouraging them, doing that silly dance, or giving high fives. Children crave our positive feedback. It's so easy to nitpick all the things that our kids struggle with, but don't miss the opportunity to celebrate each little success they have with potty training.

Teach Self-Mastery Skills

Self-mastery is taking responsibility for your own actions. Whether it's wiping, washing and drying hands, or picking out clean clothes, we can teach our children self-mastery skills that will help them be responsible for themselves. This is an invaluable life skill as an adult. We'll talk more about self-mastery in Chapter 3: Are You Ready? (page 30).

Exemplify Life Skills

Potty training gives you the opportunity to show your child that you are someone who is safe and willing to teach them essential life skills. Can you imagine how a skill like that might play out in adolescence? What if your 10-year-old is offered drugs or alcohol and feels comfortable asking you how to respond? This can even be as simple as your child feeling safe enough to ask you what a certain word means before starting to use it. The benefits of your child navigating through life with you as their guide are clear.

Set the Tone

Did you ever play a game with your parent? I remember playing very, very long games of Monopoly as a child, and the tone was very different depending on whose team I was on. If I was on a team with one of my sisters, it was full of laughs and giggles. Other relatives were focused on strategy and winning. Playing with my mom was all about teaching and encouragement. Those memories are ingrained in me: They caused me to realize what people cared about. Potty training is an opportunity for you, as the parent, to set the tone you'd like to have with your child in the long term. You get to be the one to journey along with your child to reach a goal and celebrate together.

Long-Term Motivation

Every family, and potentially even each parent within a couple, may choose to motivate differently. We'll talk in detail in Chapter 5: Your Child, Your Choice (page 72) about methods of motivation. For now, just note that you have the opportunity to choose how to motivate your child, both now and in the future.

So many parents I have helped are just fearful of what they don't know. They feel like they don't know when to start, how to start, what to do, how to handle accidents, and everything else that comes up when you

CONNECT WITH US

For a quick and free quiz to help you determine your family's "pottying personality" and navigate the process, take our three-minute quiz here: www.thepottyschool.com/quiz

Come join thousands of other parents on this journey with you! Our online support group is a place to be encouraged and lend a listening ear to others. www.facebook.com/groups /PottyTrainingSupportGroup

start to potty train your child. This book will guide you through those questions and more. You're not on your own anymore . . . you have a secret potty training weapon at your side!

I'll guide you through the five basic stages of potty training in Chapter 4: The 5-Step Potty Training Plan (page 50) and from there you can detour as needed to the special sections about issues that you may encounter. No more late-night Google searches. This book will give you a plan, remedies for issues you may encounter, and a healthy dose of confidence.

WHERE THIS PLAN COMES FROM

You don't have to take my word for it. I've had the pleasure of helping thousands of parents throughout the world via The Potty School and our online Potty Training Support Group. Whether through online or in-person classes, seminars, group speaking events, phone chat consultations, video chat consultations, or in-home consultations, there are plenty of people who have used this system with success.

In fact, we'll be hearing from some real-life parents throughout the book who have been on the journey along with me or are currently in the midst of potty training. Case studies will give you even more insight into the ins and outs of this plan, and examples of how the plan can be adjusted to fit the needs of your specific family and child.

I will cite medical studies on potty training throughout this text. Along with journal articles, medical reviews, and mommy blogs, the detailed information in this book often comes firsthand from my interactions with real parents with real potty training issues.

Choices That You Can Make

There are many different potty training choices that you get to make as a parent. It's wonderful to have that freedom, but it can be overwhelming to make these choices on your own. This book will guide you through the decision-making process. Soon you'll have your family's answers to these potty training dichotomies:

- Training Method: Naked or Garment
- Supplies: Eco-Friendly or Ease-Minded
- Motivation: Extrinsic or Intrinsic
- When to Start: Born Ready or "Wait Until They're Ready" . . . or Wait Until You're Ready

The American Academy of Pediatrics recognizes that "toilet mastery is a truly developmental milestone in a child's life." It is about a child confronting and reacting to external pressures and developing self-esteem. This can be one of the most difficult phases of development for both children and parents. That's why I'm here, to help you succeed in this difficult phase. I love encouraging parents and giving them the tools and resources necessary to teach their children. A little love and encouragement go a long way with children and parents, too!

THE 10 THINGS TO CONSIDER BEFORE YOU START

1. YOU CAN WAIT UNTIL YOUR CHILD IS READY, BUT YOU DON'T HAVE TO. Of course, we don't want to force our babies to walk when they can't even sit up, but is that actually comparable to taking off a diaper that we put them in? Take a quick look around the animal kingdom: You'll see that nearly every mammal eats, sleeps, plays, and hunts in a different location than it does its business. You don't need to feel compelled to wait because of cultural misconceptions. According to the *New York Times*, in 1957, 92 percent of one-and-a-half-year-old children were potty trained. How did we get to the place where we think we have to wait on children to be ready? It's an interesting history that we'll discuss more in Chapter 2: Is Your Child Ready? (page 13).

2. YOU CAN USE EITHER EXTRINSIC (EXTERNAL) OR INTRINSIC (INTERNAL) MOTIVATION WITH THIS PLAN. There's not only one way to motivate a child. There are best practices for both extrinsic and intrinsic rewards. Chapter 5: Your Child, Your Choice (page 72) will discuss both options in more detail.

3. YOU CAN NAKED TRAIN OR GARMENT TRAIN. Potty training while your child is naked can be a quick start to learning when your child starts going and allows you to react in real time. You can also train with your child's clothing on, though sometimes your reactions to accidents may be a bit delayed. Sometimes this delay can mean it takes a bit longer for your child to make the association you want them to make. Either way, you'll get them potty trained in the end.

4. YOU CAN BE ECO-MINDED OR EASE-MINDED. You can choose whatever you would like: paper towels or reusable cloths, a biodegradable potty or a plastic potty. The choice is yours, and the basic plan will not be altered based on your environmental or ease-based preferences.

For supply suggestions, check out check out Tools of the Trade in chapter 3 (page 34).

5. THIS PLAN ASSUMES THAT YOU HAVE THE ABILITY TO STAY HOME FOR AT LEAST ONE FULL DAY (IDEALLY THREE IN A ROW) WITH YOUR CHILD. Does that mean you'll never go out of the house? Absolutely not! However, some focused time helping your child achieve potty training success is expected. This can be a true bonding experience. Look forward to this individualized time and cherish the togetherness of you and your little one.

6. YOUR CHILD NEEDS TO BE ABLE TO COMMUNICATE, BUT IT DOESN'T HAVE TO BE VERBALLY. Some children are speech delayed and are not able to communicate with words—this plan is still for them! As long as your child can communicate with you in some way, you will be ready to get started. If your child is able to receive information and has basic comprehension, you can adapt this plan to your child. Instead of using full sentences, you'll need to break down your instruction into more basic parts of speech. You'll be mostly using action words and nouns (e.g., "go," "help," "potty," "bathroom," "toilet"). If your child is able to communicate expressively with basic hand motions, facial expressions, or other bodily motions (pointing up, reaching for Mama, or motioning to the door for "out"), these are signs that they are communicating. Generally speaking, those are all the expressive communication skills they need to tell you they need to potty. You can find more about this in Chapter 11: Special Circumstances (page 125).

7. YOU SHOULD WANT TO DO THIS. You don't have be excited to potty train per se, but you need to be leaning toward the positive side. You should see the value in teaching your child to learn to use the potty and you need to show your little one that you want to do this.

8. BEFORE YOU EVEN START, CONVINCE YOURSELF THAT IT WILL WORK THE FIRST TIME. Kids can sense fear from a mile away. If you aren't confident in their ability to succeed and in your ability to lead them, they won't be

confident, either. If you give off a sense of "we'll just take our time" or "of course there will be accidents," you'd be amazed at how much more likely they are to take their time and to have accidents. They need you to be confident. We'll talk about this in Chapter 3: Are You Ready? (page 30).

9. YOU NEED TO BE WILLING TO GUIDE THE PROCESS. When you start is up to you, but once you start, you are the leader. Take your child's needs into consideration, but understand that you are the one leading the journey. It's too much pressure to put on your child to lead this process. You need to show them that you are supportive and helpful; they have never done anything like this before.

10. YOU CAN DO THIS! Maybe you started this book thinking you have no clue where to start, how to start; what if this, or what if that? Now you have a guide to answer all those questions and more. You can be confident in your ability to potty train well from the beginning, knowing that you're using a process that is tried and true. Let's get started.

TWO

Is Your Child Ready?

Maybe it's the loads of peed-on laundry that you're sick of washing. Perhaps it's the call you got from the preschool reminding you that your child needs to be potty trained before starting, or the dreaded threat that they can't come back if they have one more accident. Maybe it's just that you're sick of messes and want to be D-O-N-E with diapers. No matter the reason, the first question you're probably asking yourself is, "How do I know when my child is ready?" You are not alone; that's the number one question that I'm asked.

In this chapter, we'll go over signs that your child is ready to be potty trained and red flags for circumstances where it would be best to wait. Potty training is not about pushing children or parents too far emotionally; it's about determining what your child is ready for so that you have reasonable expectations. In this chapter, you'll learn:

- What we mean by potty training
- How diaper training affects potty training
- How culture affects what you think is a normal age to start potty training
- What your child is feeling about parting with their diaper
- Reasonable expectations of what your child is capable of

- Red flags for some unusual circumstances where you might wait to potty train
- Answers from real parents about their potty training experiences

Let's begin by defining what potty training is. Potty training is teaching a child who was either partly or fully dependent upon diapers to stop using them and to use a socially acceptable receptacle instead.

The basic idea of potty training is shown in the flowchart on the facing page.

With the widely accepted American idea that parents should "wait until children are ready," the average age of a potty-trained child in the United States is 35 to 39 months old. By contrast, most of the world's children are potty trained by the age of one. Disposable diapers were introduced to the American market in the late 1950s; according to Andrea Olson, author of *Go Diaper Free*, it was also at that time that the potty training age of completion in the United States soared.

IS MY CHILD READY?

Do you remember when your child was a bitty baby and as soon as you took off the diaper, your kiddo started peeing or continued that explosive poop? Mammals aren't used to having their pee and poo toted around with them, so naturally as soon as kids are given the chance for their "parts" to get some air, sometimes they release. Even if you don't see signs of your child being ready to potty train, it may be that they have been so properly trained into diapers that those signs have been trained out of them. You were so effective at diaper training; I know you can be just as successful at potty training.

Think of it this way: The three-year-old who screams and demands a diaper once potty training has begun can learn to potty without complaint after time. We have trained babies to be comfortable and compliant while having a diaper on. Now, we're just doing the opposite. It helps to think of potty training as "un-diaper training."

THE STAGES OF POTTY TRAINING

WEARS DIAPERS/PULL-UPS ALL THE TIME

Wears diapers/Pull-Ups
part of the time

Doesn't wear
diapers/Pull-Ups at all

LEARNING CURVE, MAY HAVE ACCIDENTS

AWAKE TRAINED: Effectively uses a proper receptacle and stays
dry during awake hours, without accidents

DAY TRAINED: Effectively uses a proper receptacle and stays dry
during awake hours and during naps, without accidents

FULLY POTTY TRAINED: Effectively uses a proper receptacle and
stays dry during awake hours, during naps, and throughout the
night, without accidents

WHAT CULTURE DO YOU MOST IDENTIFY WITH?

Culture may be the most influential factor in what you think is a normal potty training age. According to *Diapering Habits: A Global Perspective*, "cultural norms greatly influence the age at which a baby begins toilet training." In countries that predominately use cloth diapers, such as India and China, potty training tends to begin before babies are one year old. Although Russian parents primarily use disposable diapers, they, too, practice early potty training. In countries such as Germany, France, the United Kingdom, Japan, and the United States, parents tend to wait to potty train until about two years of age. Obviously, each individual family is different, but here are the researched average ages of potty training start ages:

Countries that start potty training at 0 to 12 months:

- Kenya (4 to 5 months)
- Vietnam (9 months)
- China (before age 1)
- India (before age 1)
- Russia (before age 1)
- United States (12 months, in the years 1920 to 1940)

Countries that start potty training at 13 to 24 months:

- Palestine (14 to 15 months)
- Iran (ages 1 to 2)
- United States (18 months, in the years 1940 to 1960)

Countries that start potty training at 2 years or older:

- Germany
- France
- Japan
- United Kingdom
- United States (2 years, in the years 1960 to 1980)
- United States (2.5 years, in the years 1980 to 1990)
- United States (3 years, 1990 to present)

WHEN SHOULD *WE* START POTTY TRAINING?

We'll get to details of when you're ready to start potty training in Chapter 3: Are You Ready? (page 30), but I want to encourage you to potty train *when you want to*. Here are some common reasons that people in my potty training support group chose to start potty training exactly when they did:

- Had a few days off from work in a row
- Preschool deadline was coming up (this is a very motivating reason!)
- Child was "suspended" from preschool for too many accidents
- Waited until returning from a road trip or international trip
- Wanted the child to be potty trained before the holidays
- It was part of a New Year's resolution
- Were sick of hearing their mother-in-law talk about how young their spouse was when he was out of diapers (no joke, this has motivated several mamas I know!)

These are all fine reasons for choosing when you'd like to potty train. The secret to getting started is as easy as selecting a date and making it happen. Even if you have an ideal of "waiting for your child to be ready," "wanting it done by a certain date," or "wanting it to be child-led," all of those rationales still require you to mark a date on the calendar and stick to it. In the wise words of Benjamin Franklin, "if you fail to plan, you are planning to fail." Don't focus on your child being ready or not. You are the one to determine when this process starts.

You should brainstorm three dates where you have at least one full day (preferably two or three days in a row) to focus on potty training. Talk with your co-parent about it, calendar it, and start planning!

There are various ways to evaluate a child's readiness, but as we learned above, so much of the idea of readiness has to do with culture. It's not fair to compare a three-year-old who has never actually sat on a toilet or watched a grown-up going potty to a six-month-old who has been held over the toilet multiple times a day. If your child can tell you when they

WHAT IS YOUR CHILD FEELING ABOUT POTTY TRAINING?

Nothing. Blunt enough? To be perfectly honest, your child probably doesn't emotionally feel much of anything about potty training. You're the one worrying, not them.

Diapers, however, are a whole separate issue. That diaper is the only thing that they have had since Day One. The blankie, pacifier, breast, bottle . . . all of those things come and go, even if only for a few hours at a time. But that diaper is nearly a part of them.

Most of the time your child is perfectly happy with a diaper on—kind of like being warm and cozy in bed on a cold day. Maybe the diaper gets wet, but it's warm, so it's not so bad. Maybe there's poop, but that poop has nowhere else to go, so they get used to it. When your kiddo is wearing a diaper, it also means special time with Mommy or Daddy. Diaper changes may be the most bonding time your child has with you or a caregiver. They get focused, one-on-one attention, eye contact, and physical contact.

It's important to keep in mind that the love of their diaper has little to do with potty training and more to do with being used to the way things are and loving the one-on-one attention.

need to "go," can walk to the potty and sit down on it, and imitates your behavior, isn't that child already potty trained? And if they are able to do all of that without your help, wouldn't they have been able to accomplish at least some of it a lot sooner if you had lovingly taught them along the way?

That said, if you are waiting for these signs without actually potty training, you may have a long road of diapering ahead of you. The signs of readiness people "require" before teaching to use the potty vary from absolutely nothing to checklists based on physical, behavioral, and emotional readiness. It's interesting to note who writes such guidelines. Articles recommending a long wait are often sponsored or endorsed by diaper companies, which obviously benefit financially from long-term diaper use.

QUIZ: WHAT IS MY CHILD READY FOR?

Did your child as a baby ever finish peeing or pooping as soon as you took off their diaper?

Trick question! Most children, if changed before their next urine cycle, will release when their diaper is taken off. They naturally want to push that pee and poo away from their bodies. If you've never seen this happen, you may have been catching them just after they urinated. If you have a little one, try changing their diaper at a time you know that it will be dry, but soon before it will be wet. For those under the age of one, it will be less than an hour, maybe as little as 15 to 20 minutes, between cycles. For those ages 2 and up, it will generally be at least one to two hours.

Can your child say "up," "down," or "bye"?

If you answered yes, you can expect them to start sounding out "pee pee" or "poo poo." If you answered no, incorporating sound association aspects of elimination communication (see page 24) into your process will help immensely.

Can your child walk or crawl?

If you answered yes, they might crawl or walk to wherever you place the potty (within a reasonable distance) when you begin training. If you answered no, you can either wait on their physical development or decide that you'd like to potty train despite their inability to independently get to the potty.

If your child has a physical disability, you can decide whether you'd like to keep diapering your child in the long term. If not, you can commit to tracking your child's elimination habits over the course of several days to a week. This means logging information such as how much liquid they drank, and how long after they ate or drank that they peed or pooed. You may even want to get as specific as fiber intake if your child is nonverbal as well. You will also want to consider whether time spent doing naked observation is reasonable in your situation and if caregivers would be willing to partake as well. Special-needs children require a little more creativity, but quite often are giving off more signs of their toileting habits than we give them credit for.

Has your child shown interest in something like a doll or a new toy that they have _not_ had since infancy?

If you answered yes, that's great! This is a wonderful time to get them excited about something new: the potty! If not given the opportunity to become interested in the potty or toilet from a young age, it often doesn't naturally occur, which can lead to children being afraid of the potty, resistance, and pushback. As long as you're not overbearing and invasive of their space, bringing the potty in as a normal item in their sight and knowledge will help them be interested in this new process, possibly even sooner than you yourself feel ready! Children can then learn to be excited about and interested in other parts of the pottying process as well, like picking out new underwear and learning new skills. It's all in how you contextualize it. Make potty training feel useful for them. If you answered no, your potty training experience may be a bit more difficult. You may first want to focus on helping your child positively recognize new experiences and objects before introducing potty training into the mix.

Has your child ever hidden to go poop or pee?

If you answered yes, this is a telltale sign that your child is ready to start using the potty. Unfortunately, so many parents toss this natural occurrence aside. Since children haven't yet been taught where the poo and pee should go, it's reasonable that they don't yet "get it." If your child is hiding while pooping, they are asking for privacy; you can expect them to be able to learn that privacy can, and should, be given while in a bathroom. If you answered no, some children become so trained into diapers that they become comfortable with their own waste in their diaper. Sometimes they even expect it to be there, so if a parent tries to trick a child into potty training by cutting a hole in their diaper, the child might pitch a fit.

Does your child grab their parts before they need to go or do a "pee pee dance"?

If your child is doing these actions, it will be very helpful in teaching them an association between what they're doing and what to do about it. Many children will physically squirm and grab themselves before they go. Whether they realize what is happening can be a separate issue, one that you can teach. It is very reasonable to expect them to tell you that they need to potty ahead of when they actually go. Some children who can speak actually prefer to sign because they are so focused on the feeling of needing to pee that they can't focus on talking. For speech-delayed children, sometimes excessive signing does more harm than good, so please speak to your speech pathologist about when to use signs or not. If your child isn't physically indicating that they have to use the bathroom in an obvious way, they may never do so. Some will walk in another room, or hide behind a door, curtain, or couch. Some will be so into their play that they hardly notice going themselves, let alone stop to make a big deal about the whole thing. All of the above are totally normal.

Does your child squat to poop?

There's a reason that the Squatty Potty exists. It even exists for kids (SquattyPottymus). It is designed to mimic the body's most natural defecating position: squatting. If your child is squatting, that's a good sign that they know something is happening in their body and are trying to get it out. Squatting is a great sign that they can start telling you that they feel something happening, or can start moving to doing this on a potty or toilet. If your child isn't squatting, don't sweat it. Many children never squat and they learn to poop just fine. You just may need to teach them to sit down on the toilet before they start to poop.

RED FLAGS

Please be sensitive in your potty training timing to major life events that would affect your child's eating or bowel habits. We're not talking about moving or starting preschool. Instead, you should be aware of things like a sickness, an upcoming medical procedure or surgery, or any major physical or emotional trauma.

Odd Bowel Habits

If your child comes down with diarrhea during your training and isn't able to get to the bathroom in time, consider putting your child in diapers, even if it's only for a few days. If you are concerned that they will lose the "dry feeling" of underwear, this is one of the few times that I'd recommend putting a diaper over top of underwear. If the diarrhea is MiraLAX-induced, talk to your physician about lowering the dosage or potentially stopping the dosing altogether until things normalize a bit.

We will go into more detail on this in Chapter 6: Pooping and Peeing (page 80). Whether it's diarrhea or constipation, if your child experiences anything out of the range of "normal" bowel movements, talk to your doctor about your potty training plans.

Upcoming Medical Procedures

Take into strong consideration any medical treatment your child is undergoing. I always like to encourage parents to trust their intuition about timing when it comes to medical issues. If your child is set for surgery in two weeks, now is probably not the time to start potty training. It's highly likely that any sort of hospitalization will require the child to be put back into diapers for the sake of hospital sanitation. If your child is undergoing any ongoing medicine-based therapy, make sure you're aware of any possible side effects. With any ongoing treatments, from steroid treatments to chemotherapy, please be informed and aware and take into consideration the overall impact on your family that adding another change into life may bring.

Major Physical or Emotional Trauma

Serious trauma isn't something that's going to be forgotten overnight. You might run into a lot of issues if you are trying to potty train a child immediately after something traumatic happens to their body. If you think this may be a problem, you can seek help 24/7 from the ChildHelp National Child Abuse Hotline. Contact information is in the Resources section at the back of this book.

FAQ

I think my child is able, but I don't really know if they are ready. How can I tell if they are ready?

Make sure you go through the checklist earlier in this chapter and evaluate yourself based on your own cultural context. Also check out the Ask a Parent section at the end of this chapter for signs that other parents used to help determine when to start.

I know in other countries they start potty training as early as birth; isn't it emotionally damaging to start potty training *too early*?

Not necessarily. Here are some things I would like you to keep in mind as we start this journey:

- It is never too early to normalize the potty.
- It is never too early to start planning.
- It is never too early to point out that animals don't wear diapers.
- It is never too early for a child to see a parent using the toilet in a healthy manner and safe environment.

Baby potty training from 0 to 18 months is often called elimination communication. At its core, elimination communication is basically a form of infant hygiene. It's also used as a method of communication between child and caregiver.

Generally speaking, a sound association is created based on a parent's observations of bodily signals or based on timing to cue when the child may eliminate. This has little to do with emotions and more to do with basic sanitation and communication. There is debate over whether it is medically damaging to start potty training "too early" or "too late." There is medical research to support both options, especially if you look worldwide. That said, you may want to take into consideration the impact that diapering is having on your family's time, finances, and eco-footprint.

My child's preschool requires them to be potty trained. I don't feel like they are ready. Should I "force" them to potty train even though I don't think they are ready?

If you really feel like you don't want to potty train your child yet, I'd suggest looking for a different preschool or caring for them yourself, if possible. Day care situations like preschool require "all hands on deck" for many lessons, stations, and playground time. It simply may be that your preschool doesn't have extra hands built in to help with diaper changes. The question of whether to "force" your child is a matter of opinion. Is teaching a three-year-old to ride a bike with training wheels forcing them to learn? Some would say yes, some would say no. Keep in mind that a family member might view potty training not as forcing but as teaching, and choose to teach your child while you're away. If you don't want to train your child out of diapers, and you don't have other preschool options, then preschool might not be the best fit right now for your family.

My child hides in a corner to poop. Does that mean they're ready to potty train?

This is a child asking for privacy, which is a good thing. It is a great indicator that they're ready to learn where privacy can, and should, be given: in the bathroom. For more details about hiding and pooping, refer to Chapter 6: Pooping and Peeing (page 80).

I think my child is ready, and has already shown success. But when I take them to preschool, a family member's house, or babysitter's house, someone always puts a diaper on them. How do I explain that they are able to be out of diapers?

Don't argue. Don't rationalize. Don't explain. Just show other people your child's success. Seeing is believing. If your child had a full day of success at home, then tell caregivers that. If your child stays dry during awake hours, but needs a diaper for a nap, say so. The more communication of facts, the better. Arrive a few minutes early to wherever you're going and take your child to the bathroom yourself when you first get there (preferably in the same location that the child will typically be using there, if possible). When other caregivers see you having success, they will want to follow suit.

I don't think my child understands what potty training is and they don't seem interested. Should I just wait?

Unless we're talking about a cognitive delay, your child probably understands the basic concept that "pee and poo go in the potty" if you have explained it and shown it to them one or two times. Now, transferring that to actions is a different story. If the child is old enough to show to you that they have chosen to be uninterested, even after explanation, you could hold off to get your own bearings, or you could stop talking about potty training and just start it. If you're asking this because your child has had a lot of accidents, then you should try naked-from-the-waist-down time so that you can immediately take them when they start going. That will make the clearest, fastest association for them.

How can I get my stubborn toddler to potty train? They don't want to wear diapers but want to pee standing up wherever they are!

If your child is peeing wherever they are, as soon as they start peeing, you should take them to the potty. Don't let them pee on your carpet or floor! As soon as they start, take them by the hand and walk them to the bathroom. Even if they pitch a fit, bring them with you. Even if you only get a few drops into the potty, that counts as a success. You'll probably surprise them and stop the flow of urine the first time, but you know there's more in there. That means sometime soon they'll need to go again, and you'll be ready to walk them over to the potty.

If peeing standing up is an issue, you could always have your child go in the shower. If your child has sensory processing disorder or is autistic, they could be extra sensitive to how things feel. You could also give them the option to kneel on the toilet. Or maybe the simple difference of sitting

Ask a Parent

How did you know your child was ready, even if everyone else thought you were crazy?

"She was telling me that her diaper needed to be changed. Telling me she went poop." —DIANA

"Took off her diaper and gave me a clean one at 18 months. My older one would bring me to the bathroom and take her diaper off. At that time, she was about a year old! We also had her on the potty since she was three months. She'd wake up with a dry diaper." —CHRIS

"Enough was enough on my end as a parent! My encouragement and not giving up even through the toughest situations. It showed her that she can do it! I'm her biggest fan! And she loves to make me cheer! Going potty is one of my biggest cheers!" —LUANNA

"My little one started hiding to go poop and started waking up dry in the mornings." —ASHLEY

"My 20-month-old daughter was able to follow simple commands. For example, we would sing a song that said, 'Pointer finger up. Put it on your head,' and she would do the motions while singing the song. It was very basic, but I knew there was some understanding of commands and a desire to please me. She didn't really talk a lot, but what she lacked in verbal communication she made up for nonverbally in that she would smile at me when she was happy or run to the door when I said, 'Daddy is home!' To me, her ability to communicate nonverbally was sufficient and I didn't need her to tell me she had to go potty with words as long as she could physically run to the potty when needed." —HOPE

on the toilet facing the tank will make them feel more secure and solve the problem.

Maybe the joy of flushing when they're done will encourage them to sit down so they can watch it more closely. Or maybe you'll learn that they don't like all the sounds and are trying to distance themselves as much as possible. Try to not only fix the situation, but figure out what your child is trying to tell you through their behavior.

How do I determine if my child is truly not ready or if they're just making a choice?

Rely on your intuition for this one. A good trick is to test if your child displays stubborn behavior about other actions you are requiring of them. Are they pushing back on helping put away stuffed animals? Are they yelling "no" at the drop of a hat? This may indicate a behavioral stage that isn't directly related to the ability to learn to use the potty.

I tried potty training previously and it didn't go well because they weren't ready. How do I ensure that they're ready this time?

First off, are *you* ready? Whether your child is ready or not doesn't matter if you aren't ready to train them. Take a quick introspective look at whether you're willing to lead them. Sometimes the biggest test for this is, "Would I want to learn how to use the potty from me, right now?"

Once you yourself are set, you have a plan, and you have reasonable expectations for your child's success, then you can expect success. I would encourage you to ensure that they're ready this time by doing as much prep ahead of time as possible. Talk about how normal using the potty is; point the bathroom out in stores. Make their favorite bedtime-story characters need to go potty before bed—anything to make pottying seem normal to them. The more normal it is to your child, the easier it will be to incorporate it into their regular routine once you are ready to lead them.

I feel like this whole potty training thing has become an emotional struggle, more than physical. Why is that?

Before a certain age (about 13 to 18 months) the only attachment your child has to a diaper is physical. Once they start getting emotionally attached, though, potty training becomes a whole different ball game. Some kids love a diaper like they love a lovey, a blankie, or a beloved stuffed animal. Taking away a beloved item from a child can be emotionally trying, but it's like ripping off a Band-Aid: Often, faster is less painful than slow removal.

A Note from Jennifer Singer, MD

When a child should be toilet trained is controversial. In general, I advise parents that their child should demonstrate emotional readiness and the achievement of adequate motor skills before being trained. According to the American Academy of Pediatrics, training too early can create undue stress that may delay the very process that is being trained. In the United States, many medical professionals advocate a recommended training start age of 18 to 24 months with the normal process occurring through about age 3½. The Centers for Disease Control suggest that toilet training is a behavioral milestone and should be complete by age 5. While training can be done earlier, as is evidenced by international data and supported in this book, doing so before a child can proficiently walk or climb to the toilet can carry risks if not properly executed. If you wish to try to train your child before 18 months of age, please keep in mind these normal bladder-emptying cycles when setting expectations for your child to reach the toilet in time:

- Up to 6 months voiding occurs hourly
- 6 to 12 months voiding occurs every 1½ to 2 hours
- 13 months to 24 months voiding occurs about every 2½ hours

THREE

Are You Ready?

YOU'RE THE LEADER

You get to be the head, director, CEO, manager, or captain of pottying! Maybe it sounds overwhelming, but think of it from your child's perspective. It's like they're standing waiting to get picked on a team and they're just hoping you'll pick them, to coach them and teach them. And then you do and their little heart does a happy dance. Yes, you can call yourself the "Potty Boss," but you don't get to be bossy! You get to be the leader who:

- Encourages
- Knows what they need even before they do
- Guides them each step of the way

I don't mean to overly focus on this, but can you imagine how great that must be to a little kid? What a sense of comfort and encouragement that must bring to know that you are going to be there for them. Even if there are setbacks outside of your care, you'll be there to help guide them.

A child who is super excited by anything new in their world gets the chance to learn, from one of their favorite people, how to do something that might be a bit scary to them. You are the perfect person for the job! It might be tough, but stay positive! Your child isn't trying to personally attack you; they are just questioning the change.

WHEN TO BE FIRM BUT FAIR

Situations will arise when you'll need to be firm, but fair. Think of these scenarios:

- You told your child no more diapers, but they pitch a fit when you try to take it off. (Hint: Take the diaper off first.)
- They pee on the floor right after you say, "Pee pee goes in the potty." (Hint: Have them wait and "help" you clean up in some way.)
- They want to sit on the couch, but you say, "No naked bottoms on the couch." (Hint: Lay a waterproof mat down if you want to compromise.)
- They want to wear undies at preschool, but they're having multiple accidents a day at home. (Hint: Use wearing undies at preschool as a "reward" for potty success at home.)
- They want to sit on the big toilet, but you're afraid that they'll fall off if you're not there. (Hint: Get a mini potty.)
- You pack up and tell them they need to go potty before you leave, and they say they don't need to go. (Hint: Go at the same time, with them on the mini potty. That way it's normal to go potty every time before you leave.)

7 Effective Strategies to Make Potty Training a Success

How do we actually become those successful, effective potty training people? Thai Nguyen's article "Success Starts with Self-Mastery: 7 Effective Strategies" is such a poignant resource for our own self-reflection, but it's equally effective in the context of leading our child's pottying journey. We'll see not only the skills but also the self-mastery that we can teach our children throughout this process.

1. TALK TO YOURSELF POSITIVELY: Can you imagine if every time you doubted your ability to do something you had already been trained to think, "I can do this! What's the next best step to take?" We can teach our children to have a positive voice in their head, a "yes, I can do this" voice. This is a huge life skill!

2. MAKE PEACE WITH YOUR PAST: This is one we can all learn from, but for the sake of potty training we can be the ones to teach our littles to forgive themselves for any accidents and move on to their next opportunity to succeed.

3. PLAY DEVIL'S ADVOCATE: Confronting yourself and coming at your requests from another's perspective—in this case, your child's perspective—can do wonders in encouraging graciousness with other human beings.

4. KEEP A JOURNAL: In this case, we can be keeping a tracker. It will help us see where we've been, which will help us determine where we're going, and on which path.

5. BREAK THE BYSTANDER EFFECT: If you're at a friend's house for a dinner party and a child starts grunting at the table, obviously pooping, the more people that are there, the less likely any one person is to take responsibility—that is, unless a self-mastered person is there willing to jump into action where action is needed. We want to teach our children to be this way, too. We don't just want them noticing they need

to potty; we want them to be the one who springs into action to do something about it. It doesn't sound like a truly heroic act when we're talking about potty training, but as a life skill it is one that is lacking in our society.

6. PRACTICE COGNITIVE REAPPRAISAL: Are you able to reevaluate a situation to see the silver lining? Can you find the good in a bad situation? Would you be able to look at a child who just pooped in their crib and wiped it on the wall, and have the ability to notice that they yelled out to you, "Mama, I pooped," and see that as an actual step toward potty learning? This is a teachable skill we can help our children master.

7. AUDIT YOURSELF: In order to succeed, we need to be able to admit the skills that need improving. We can help teach our children that they can still have pottying success, even if they need to ask for help with their pants or with turning off the water. Take some time to audit your child's (and your own) capabilities and things that they still have room to grow in, and accept that as part of the learning process.

Be an encouraging, reasonable parent who truly wants to help your child. They will sense that. Do your best to stay consistent.

YOU CAN MAINTAIN YOUR GROUND BY DOING A FEW THINGS:

- Don't give in just because your child asks.
- Don't grab a diaper just because they're throwing a fit; you'll teach them that they get what they want when they throw a fit. They are adjusting. Stick with what you said.
- Restate what you said and ask your child if they understand. Then, have them reply while giving you eye contact.
- Be consistent. Say what you'll do. Then do what you said.
- Be willing to change. If something really isn't working, you're the parent. Talk with your co-parent, get on the same page, and then clearly reset the guidelines for your child, recognizing that things have changed and that might be hard for them.

TOOLS OF THE TRADE

While there's no substitute for good parenting, there are several products and pieces of household equipment that may be helpful throughout the pottying journey. Mind you, you can potty train with no more than a child and a receptacle of choice, but we'll assume if you're reading this book that you enjoy a few modern luxuries and would like your child to be as comfortable as possible within your means. Each family has different needs and preferences, and you may require more specialized product recommendations. For the average child, however, these are some "top picks." For a comprehensive list of tools and resources, please visit www.thepottyschool.com/tools.

Potties

BUILT-IN TOILET SEAT

Mayfair NextStep Adult Toilet Seat with Built-in Child Potty Training Seat: I wish I had a Mayfair NextStep Adult Toilet Seat with Built-in Child Potty Training Seat when I started training my first child. If you ever plan to have visitors at home or have more than one child, and you have the long-term vision in mind, a built-in potty training seat is a very worthwhile investment. Though this is the priciest of the "potty" options, the price is comparable to a box of diapers.

MINI POTTY (ALSO REFERRED TO AS A POTTY CHAIR OR TODDLER TOILET)

BabyBjörn Potty Chair / BabyBjörn Smart Potty: I love mini potties! Teaching a child to use a mini potty can be a lifesaver to a pregnant mama, a parent with a new baby, or anyone with back problems. Mini potties don't require you to pick up your child and place them on a potty. They also avoid the hassle and fall risk of using a stool.

There are two types of mini potties:

- **All-in-one option (no insert, made of one piece):** The benefit of this option is that it's one of the cheapest potties on the market. The negative is that you'll very soon find out why it's so cheap. It typically can't be easily dumped in the toilet, and rinsing it off in the sink can be a messy hassle.
- **With insert (two pieces):** The best part of this option is that it is easy to clean, and kids can often dump it into the big toilet on their own. The negatives are that kids try to dump it into the big toilet on their own (and don't always make it) and it typically can't be placed within arm's reach of the toilet paper.

The mini potty in our kids' bathroom is a **BabyBjörn Potty Chair.** This is the most durable mini potty I have found. The style without a back, called a **BabyBjörn Smart Potty**, is also wonderful. I highly recommend them both.

Helpful Hint: If you live in a cold place, your child has sensory processing disorder, or you just want to make it a bit cozier, try making a "potty cozy."

URINAL

mkool Cute Frog Potty Training Urinal for Boys: The mkool Cute Frog Potty Training Urinal for Boys is for teaching boys to urinate standing up. Anatomically, it isn't made for a girl. Urinals are the wall equivalent of mini potties. They either come as an all-in-one or have an insert to take out and rinse. I recommend the latter.

TOILET SEAT REDUCER (ALSO CALLED A TOILET TRAINER OR TOILET RING)

BabyBjörn Toilet Trainer: My favorite item for early trainers, small-bottomed kids, or kids who aren't stable enough to sit on the big potty alone is the BabyBjörn Toilet Trainer. Toilet seat reducers come in multiple options: anything from the foldable kind you can throw in your diaper bag (which I don't recommend because they can be unstable), to squishy-topped ones, to those that are adjustable and fit any toilet size. A BabyBjörn Toilet Trainer has been a part of our family's potty training supplies since Day One, and it has lasted for years.

TRAVEL POTTY

Kalencom 2-in-1 Potette Plus: Oh travel potty, how I love thee! Seriously, folks, this one is a freedom-giver! No longer will you be wishing you knew where the bathroom is in every single store you go to. This one tool has given me so much more confidence as a mom. The Kalencom 2-in-1 Potette Plus potty is my "backup diaper." It can fold up and live in the trunk of your car, in the bottom of your stroller, or even in your diaper bag. This one doubles as a seat reducer, too. If you prefer a larger potty with a lid, those are available as well. This is the travel potty our family uses nearly daily.

Step Stool

BabyBjörn Step Stool: A good, old-fashioned stool will definitely do the trick, but the added bonus of an anti-slip surface on both the top and bottom—especially when you're dealing with various liquids in the bathroom—makes the BabyBjörn Step Stool a good choice. The more chances for success in being independent that you give your child, the better.

Soap

Kandoo Foaming Hand Soap: The easier to wipe off, the better! Generally speaking, I recommend foaming soap. Your child will be washing their hands multiple times a day. With foaming or clear-colored soap, you won't be spending your afternoons wiping down a colorful, soap-splattered sink. Kandoo Foaming Hand Soap is gentle enough to use many times a day without drying out your skin.

Toilet Paper or Flushable Wipes

Charmin Ultra Soft Toilet Paper / Kandoo Kids Flushable Wipes:
There's no need to buy special toilet paper, but if you're looking for something to "enjoy the go," Charmin's Ultra Soft Toilet Paper is both durable and quite soft. If you're looking for something to take with you on the go, Kandoo Kids Flushable Wipes are perfect for the job.

Toilet Sprayer

Bumworks Cloth Diaper Toilet Sprayer Kit: A toilet sprayer comes in handy for everything from rinsing the mini potty, to cloth diapering, to rinsing out the steam-cleaning vacuum cleaner.

Undies

Tiny Undies / Gerber Training Pants / Tiny Trainers / Super Undies / TinyUps: A must-have! Get at least six to ten pairs. Many prefer 20 pairs so that they're not constantly doing laundry. For small sizes, try Tiny Undies. For training pants, you can use Gerber Training Pants or Tiny Trainers. Use Super Undies or TinyUps for out-and-about and overnight underwear.

Oversized Pants

Hanes EcoSmart Fleece Pants: We're not going for fashion; we're going for practicality. That means no zippers or buttons. Get a pair of pants that are one or two sizes too large (for ease of pulling up and pushing down), such as Hanes EcoSmart Fleece Pants.

Pajamas

PeeJamas: This exact item has been a brainchild of mine for a while, but PeeJamas beat me to the chase. They are two-piece, non-zippered, non-leaking, undies-included jammies.

Sheets

QuickZip: You will be changing sheets. You can double-layer sheets and mattress protectors, but QuickZip sheets are really simple. You just zip off the soiled sheet, wipe off the mattress protector, and zip on the new sheet. Presto!

Mattress Protector

American Baby Company Waterproof Fitted Crib and Toddler Protective Mattress Pad Cover (for crib/toddler bed) / Priva High Quality Ultra Waterproof Sheet and Mattress Protector (for co-sleeping): You need a mattress pad like the American Baby Company Waterproof Fitted Crib and Toddler Protective Mattress Pad Cover, or you'll have a very stinky, yucky mattress.

If you co-sleep, make sure to buy one that fits your bed, or just use a portable mattress pad, like the Priva High Quality Ultra Waterproof Sheet and Mattress Protector, and hope it doesn't get kicked out of the way in the night.

Faucet Extender

Prince Lionheart Faucet Extender: The Prince Lionheart Faucet Extender extends the faucet so your child can reach the water. You can also make an extender from a shampoo bottle by yourself.

Car Seat Protector

Summer Infant Deluxe Piddle Pad: Car seats are a pain to wash. When you have to go somewhere and you're waiting for a car seat to air-dry (or hoping it doesn't shrink too much in the dryer), you'll wish you had a Summer Infant Deluxe Piddle Pad. Well past the stage of fearing an accident on the way to the grocery store, you can use this for road trips or travel in the evening.

Nightlight

Suptempo LED Toilet Bowl Night Light: Your child may not be used to walking around the house at night, and that can be scary. Anything that can help minimize the scary factor, like a Suptempo LED Toilet Bowl Night Light, is of great use.

Prizes

Target's Bullseye's Playground: If you are motivating your child extrinsically (with something tangible), you'll want something to reward them with. People choose anything from food treats, to toys, to coloring books. My go-to suggestion is anything from the Bullseye's Playground section at Target.

Cleaning Supplies

STAIN REMOVER

OxiClean Versatile Stain Remover: OxiClean Versatile Stain Remover is the most effective stain remover I have ever used.

CARPET CLEANING

Nature's Miracle Pet Stain and Odor Remover Foam Aerosol Sprays: For some reason, customers always claim that dog urine products, like Nature's Miracle Pet Stain and Odor Remover, work far better than "human" odor-removing products.

DISINFECTING WIPES

Seventh Generation Disinfecting Multi-Surface Wipes / Clorox Disinfecting Wipes: Seventh Generation Disinfecting Multi-Surface Wipes are an eco-friendly wipe option. A bleach-based wipe, such as Clorox Disinfecting Wipes, is good for end-of-the-day potty training cleanup to make sure you're not spreading germs.

A PROPER ENVIRONMENT

Where Will You Potty Train?

When you are getting ready to start the potty training journey, one of the first thoughts that you have is where you are going to do it. Your "pottying space" can be anywhere you'd like. Be creative when considering your needs and availability. You may use:

- The bathroom
- The living room with a mini potty close by
- A room adjacent to a bathroom
- The kitchen, because of easy-to-clean flooring
- The backyard
- A relative's house
- A hallway connecting rooms
- A patio

ALL ABOUT UNDIES

What kind of undies should you use on a newly potty trained child?

In general, I recommend buying undies that are at least one or two sizes above your child's current garment size so that they can easily learn to push them down and pull them up on their own (and they can grow into them, too). Simple cotton, one-layer undies will do the trick. You want your child to notice the wetness on their skin and be able to see or feel that they are wet from the outside as well, so they can make the association that they made the undies wet. The more they feel the wetness and messiness, the better.

One kind of undies I used with my kiddos was Tiny Undies, because there are small sizes available (starting at 6 months, all the way to 5T), and because it is a mama-run, sustainable company. If your child's accidents are often giant puddles, you may want to start using "training" undies, like Gerber Training Pants or Tiny Trainers—instead of just one layer, these have multiple layers of cloth for more absorbance. If you happen to be running errands or going on a long car ride, or even in certain preschool day care situations, a layer over the undies can help with cleanup. TinyUps (cloth covers that go over underwear) or Super Undies (which have a thin waterproof layer) will keep outer garments dry.

Unless your child has severe special needs, I would always consider Pull-Ups a diaper, not underwear. But once you get past in-home training, the additional layers and waterproof barriers can be a big help for cleanup on the go.

Prepare the Space

You'll want to provide basic essentials in an easy-to-access way.
These should include:

- Potty or toilet
- Toilet paper or flushable wipes
- Hand soap
- Towel

Feel free to add some potty-only toys or activities, too. Just don't
make them too distracting. Remember the saying, "Start as you mean to
go on." If you don't want your child using electronics while they're on the
toilet in the long term, don't start that way.

FOR THE SAKE OF SANITATION:

- Move any carpets and rugs out of your potty training space.
- Plan to have lots of clean rags on hand.
- Be prepared for some mess—if you know it will bother you,
  get some rubber gloves.
- Have extra laundry detergent and stain remover on hand.
- Have disinfectant wipes easily accessible.
- Fill the steam cleaner the night before so it's ready.

THE READINESS CHECKLIST

Are You Ready to Potty Train?

So, are you ready to do this? Below are the things you need to have lined
up to be ready for potty training. All of them are prerequisites and none
of them are optional.

- ☐ You have a potty training plan personalized to your child and
  your family.

☐ You know that there will be ups and downs, but you're ready to teach your child with a good attitude!

☐ You have any supplies purchased and actually on hand (a mini potty, travel seat reducer, undies, etc.).

☐ You have a potty training buddy: someone you can check in with and seek helpful advice from along the way, even if it's a virtual buddy. (You might think this should be optional, but you'll be glad of your buddy if you end up with a rough first day.)

☐ You have prepared to reduce your other responsibilities as much as possible during potty training (things like meal preparation, other children's care, work, and volunteering).

FAQ

I'm just afraid I'm going to mess this all up. How do I avoid ruining my child's potty training experience?

This is so incredibly normal. How could you possibly feel confident in something you've never done before? Parenting is such a trip. It's as though as soon as you're ready and feel confident in one stage, it's already over.

Think back to that first tooth and figuring out how to ease teething pain. How overwhelmed did you feel? How much Internet searching did you do? It's okay if you don't feel ready. You probably won't ever feel fully ready for something you haven't done before. Sometimes you just have to trust yourself a little bit more than you feel comfortable with. You can do this. You'll need some help along the way, but that's not a reason to not start. Children learn so incredibly well from their parents and guardians; anything you have to offer them in guidance will go much further than it will from anyone else in their lives. They trust you. They love you. Just remember that.

There are so many changes happening in life; should I wait until life calms down a bit?

There are no guarantees that life will ever calm down. That said, if you earnestly see an end in sight to the crazies that are causing you undue stress, then by all means, wait. A few weeks one way or another won't be a big deal in the scheme of life. Waiting a few months is a much bigger deal and I'd suggest more caution in waiting that long. If you're not in a good place emotionally or you're feeling highly stressed, it's a pretty good bet that you won't be the most effective teacher. Consider it this way: Has your child ever been around you with this level of stress before? If so, give it a go. If not, maybe set yourself a reminder for a week and then reevaluate. Things may have changed drastically in a week.

We're moving. Is now a good time to start potty training?

There are so many variables to consider; I wish I knew what yours were! Are you moving across the state? To the next street? To another country? If you're willing to keep your pottying accessories within arm's length and you have help with packing and unpacking, then you certainly can start whenever you'd like. If you're on your own driving across the country, that's a bit different. It's mostly a matter of your level of distraction. I don't typically encourage setting an alarm, but it may be useful to set one just to make yourself take potty breaks. Moving doesn't seem to be an overly traumatic event that a child can't move past and adapt to. The biggest thing is making sure they know how to get to the new bathroom!

I'm pregnant! Should I potty train now or after the baby comes?

Congratulations! I'm so happy for you and your new little life! How far along are you? How sick are you feeling? Do you have someone to help you with your older child once the baby comes? Do you have a mini potty? I wish I could grab a cup of coffee with you, give you a hug, and hear how life is for you right now, then guide you from there. There's not a one-size-fits-all answer for this by any means. Generally speaking, if you're feeling mostly your normal self and you have at least a month before you expect your new baby, I'd say go for it. If you're seven months pregnant, you have all-day "morning" sickness, and your back is killing you, you might want to consider waiting until after the baby comes. My basic rule of thumb is to ask your co-parent or even a best friend what they think is best for your whole family, and then decide from there.

I have a new baby, and I think my older child is regressing. Should I just put them back in diapers?

How much success have you had? Is your child able to get to the toilet on their own? Are they willing to wait for you to help them wipe if needed? Somehow people have created a notion that children regress when there's a new baby. I haven't found that to be the baby's fault. Typically, it's because the parent, who used to be extremely attentive, is now sharing that attention with a new baby. Think about it from your toddler's perspective. Think about what an attentive hawk you were regarding their every pottying move: praising their every success, helping them wash their hands. And then the baby came. Boom. Mom's calling, "If you need to potty, walk to the bathroom, please!" and "I'll be there in a minute," and "Just a second, I'm feeding the baby." It's a big change for them. Most likely they don't need diapers; they just need more time with you. I encourage you to try to sneak in some extra cuddle time by reading stories on the couch or by taking a quick nature walk, even if it's only three steps outside your front door.

Give them a little more eye contact and say more sweet things to them. You probably don't have much in you to give, but whatever you can provide will be rewarded tenfold in obedience and willingness, which helps a whole lot when you need to tell a child to sit down and wait for you to help and wipe them. Trust me.

Ask a Parent

What do you wish you knew and prepared for ahead of your potty training experience?

"I wish I would have started talking to her about it sooner rather than denying that she's ready." —DENISE

"Having help around the house." —SARAH

"Patience." —KOURTNEY

"Education on how constipation affects potty training." —MARIA

"I wish I had prepared my mattress for accidents." —KHLOE

"A manual book that came out my vagina saying, 'how to potty train them from birth,' lol." —CHRISTINE

"That my son is more interested in peeing and pooping (yes, both) outside with the dog! He just goes out there but the potty, oh my!" —AMBER

"[To] wash all my towels and have them all lined up neatly in the closet." —SUZIE

"[That] it was going to take longer than a few weeks." —JUNE

"Getting undies in my daughter's size. She's in 12–18 months. She is 18 months and small for her age. I cannot find any that fit her, all size 2T and up. The struggles of potty training young!" —CHRISTOPHER

"That we didn't move during potty time, but we had to." —TANIA

"A house with no carpet so I could keep in him in underwear instead of Pull-Ups." —REESE

"The knowledge to make my two-year-old daughter understand that we don't stand to pee and that you have to sit more than two seconds to go on the potty." —DANIELLE

"My third child. She's number 3 and number 1 got potty trained at day care, number 2 just woke up one day and started using the potty, number 3 . . . has to be a challenge." —NICOLE

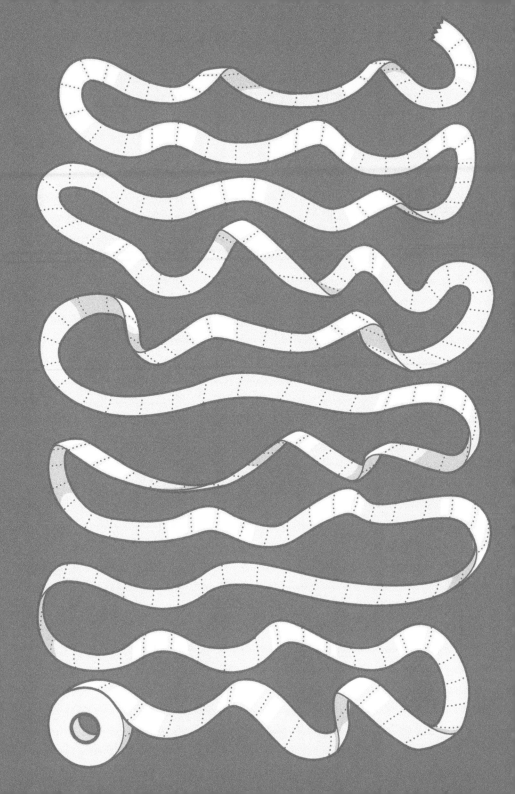

Part Two

HOW TO POTTY TRAIN YOUR CHILD

The 5-Step Potty Training Plan

Your Child, Your Choice

Pooping and Peeing

Nighttime and Napping

Out and About

Family and Other Caregivers

FOUR

The 5-Step Potty Training Plan

HOW FAST CAN I GET THIS DONE?

I'm a realist. I won't promise you that your child will be potty trained in one day. But I'm also sad for people when I hear that they have been potty training for months and months. I've even heard of people doing so for over a year. Potty training in its entirety shouldn't take more than a month for daytime, and a max of a few months for day and awake. Sometimes night training comes later and can be a separate thing altogether, depending on the child and if there are any underlying medical conditions to consider.

If you personalize this plan to your child, your family, your circumstances, and where you are in the pottying journey, it will take you anywhere from one hour to one month to start and finish (or just finish) potty training an "average" child. The average amount of time is two days to one week for daytime, and one day to one month for nighttime. Keep in mind that results may vary. Children with autism, Down syndrome, and other developmental delays *can* use this system, though their successes will look different and be more incremental.

Remember that quiz you took in chapter 2 about what your child was ready for? This is where that plays out. Here are some things to remember about expectations:

- Yes, you can expect an 18-month-old to start using the potty with reasonable success within a few days, but it is unreasonable to expect them to push down and pull up their pants and wipe on their own.
- Yes, you can expect a child with autism (who isn't used to fully emptying their bladder because they're being taken every hour) to learn what the feeling of a full bladder is and learn to start emptying it. But there will almost assuredly be some accidents during that transition.
- Yes, some can successfully potty train a child in the two days before preschool starts. But the level of stress for success you put on them and on yourself typically isn't worth the procrastination. I recommend putting in a buffer of a month or two before starting preschool or another program that requires your child to be fully potty trained.

I encourage you and your child to focus on one step at a time, rather than the entire plan all at once. Step by step, in order, we'll get there.

The goal isn't speed: The ultimate goal is accident-free potty independence. A child who is potty trained in two days, is wearing undies, but has an accident every day isn't in a better place than a child who took seven days to potty train but has no accidents. There will be ups and downs. This journey ebbs and flows. Be willing to be flexible to the changes alongside your child. Feel free to use the tracker at the back of this book to monitor your child's progress along the journey.

OPTIONAL STEP

You and Your Child: Quality Time

No one is eager to learn from someone who doesn't seem to care about them and what they care about. That said, please try to squeeze in some quality time with your child *before* you start. Remind yourself how much you love them. Try to squeeze that in.

SOME IDEAS FOR SPENDING TIME TOGETHER:

(The starred ideas can be done during the first day of potty training, too!)

- A simple game* (e.g., Candy Land, matching game)
- An art project* (e.g., a crayon leaf rubbing)
- A short walk*
- A one-on-one trip to pretty much anywhere
- A picnic dinner at a new park
- A trip to get a treat, like frozen yogurt or ice cream
- A quick stop by the pet store to visit the fish or the puppies

Let's never be too busy for quality time, for memories, and for loving and appreciating our children.

Self-Reflection

Are you in a place to be teaching your child? Sometimes it's a case of postpartum depression, sometimes it's the I-haven't-seen-the-sun-in-three-weeks blues, or sometimes you can't put your finger on it, but you're just feeling overwhelmingly like you just can't succeed as a parent. Some fresh air and nature's beauty often do the trick, but sometimes you need to give yourself a little more space and time before you add another endeavor to your plate. Here are a few questions to ask yourself, and answer yes to before starting!

DOES THIS PLAN ACTUALLY WORK?

Let's hear from some parents who have successfully gone through this program:

"I was literally crying before our conference call, I was so tired and hopeless after six days of unsuccessful potty training. After I talked to Michelle, my son never peed on the ground or in his pants again! That day he peed in the toilet every time, the next day he peed without screaming, and today he peed on a real public potty and pooped for the first time! He snuck in and pooped without us even knowing!" —MARY

"Michelle was so helpful in outlining a plan to train my twins. I was so intimidated before talking with her, and she really showed me how to move forward and bring the diaper years to an end! Thank you, Michelle!" —CATHERINE

☐ Are you of a mind-set to lovingly teach your child?

☐ Are you willing to serve your child by teaching them something new?

☐ Are you willing to humble yourself to do "menial" tasks, such as cleaning up pee and poo off the floor and clothes? (If not, do you have a plan in place for someone else to do it?)

☐ Are you willing to compromise with your co-parent to decide on the details of the plan together?

☐ Are you willing to step a bit into the unknown in order to get the job done?

STEP 1

INTRODUCE THE TOILET

I will say this over and over again. **My number one piece of advice, by far, is to make using the potty NORMAL.** If children see using the potty as a huge, new transition to something they're unfamiliar with, it can be scary and they will push back. It's like telling your child to get in the car with a complete stranger. Of course that's alarming! But if you tell them to get in the car with a neighbor with whom they are familiar, even if they've never talked to them, your child will be much more comfortable with the idea. The same goes for potty training: Build on familiarity.

Ways to Normalize the Potty

Here are a few strategies for getting your child comfortable around the toilet:

- Talk about taking a potty break and have them walk to the bathroom with you. Many children will ask to try a mini potty if it's sitting there!
- Let them watch you.
- Read pottying stories to them to teach about others who are exploring and learning about the toilet. I have suggestions in the Resources section at the back of this book.
- Give your child a tour of the bathroom. Name each component with its proper name and let them repeat after you. Then describe what each item does. "This is a mirror; you can see your reflection. This is a toilet; it's where pee pee and poo poo go."
- Give your potty a name and introduce it to your child. This can work well for children who are "scared" of the potty.
- Let your child flush the toilet on their own to experiment, but then save it for when they actually put something in the toilet.

It's not essential to the potty training process that your child know how to push down and pull up their pants before starting to potty train. Most children are able to start learning to push down and pull up pants around 18 to 24 months. That said, it might be worth teaching them how to do it *while* you're potty training. If given stretchy-waist, loose pants that are one or two sizes too big, most children at two years of age or older are able to pull up and push down their pants.

STEP 2
MAKE A CLEAN BREAK

You probably know firsthand how agonizing it can be for both a parent and a child to slowly rip off a Band-Aid. But if you rip it off quickly it can be so much less painful. Think of getting rid of diapers like that: quick and painless. Yes, you could make it a slow transitional process and it will work, but easing into it will not work as quickly and will actually not be easier on your child.

Children often think in terms of black and white and right and wrong. The simpler it is to follow, the easier it will be for them to get, so let's make it simple. According to "Cognitive Development," an article published by Cincinnati Children's Hospital, the ability to reason and think abstractly is something that doesn't even develop until adolescence.

Don't make switching from diapers to undies a days-long process. Don't switch back and forth from diapers to undies and vice versa. You can, however, tell your child ahead of time what happens when people learn to use the potty. That is part of normalizing the process.

As far as telling them you're going to take off *their* diaper, don't stretch out the process. At most, tell them the night before. Ideally, just take off the diaper the first morning of training and then tell them it's not coming back. Don't mention or show it to them again. Did you hear that? That means, **don't even say the word *diaper* while you're potty training!** No need to pour salt on a wound and potentially make things worse.

You *can* do something to mark the transition, but I wouldn't suggest having it take more than a few minutes. Here are some ideas you *could* (but definitely don't need to) try to help your child through the transition:

- "Give" unused diapers to a younger relative or friend (typically on the phone works better than in person; otherwise your child may cling to those diapers for dear life).
- Have an undies celebration to go pick out big-kid undies.
- Have them throw the last diaper in the trash, maybe even in the "big trash can" or dumpster, to mark the occasion.

Here are a few phrases that you can use when talking to your child about switching from diapers to the toilet:

- "Pee pee and poo poo go in the potty now."
- "It's only the potty now."
- "Big girls/big boys _____!" (e.g., get to go on the toilet, don't use diapers, wear undies) Please note that this one can often backfire. So be ready for the possibility of their arguing that they don't want to be "big" but prefer to stay a "baby." If that happens, just steer clear of emphasizing the "big girls/big boys" part in the future.
- (If using a diaper just for naps/night) "This is for sleeping. Just for when you rest." If possible, avoid saying "diaper" at all. But, don't call Pull-Ups or other non-wet-feeling options "undies."
- "Diapers are gone. Now, let's keep your undies 'dry dry' and put your pee pee and poo poo in the toilet."
- "I know you can put your pee/poo in the potty just like Mommy/Daddy does!"
- "Yay! You get to start using the toilet like [big brother/big sister/cousin/friend] does!"

Remember to be true to your word. After you toss the diapers, don't go back on what you said. Even if there are tantrums and fits, remember that this is better in the long term and even in the short term! If you give in to a fit or tantrum now and let them have control over the situation, then you are teaching your child to throw fits in order to control how you act as a parent and the guidelines that you set for them.

Stay strong! You can do this. After a few days, possibly even a few hours, fits like this will be a thing of the past.

STEP 3
HYDRATE AND OBSERVE

It is so helpful to have as many opportunities as possible to teach kids where to put that pee and poo. Being hydrated gives you just that. Keeping your child hydrated is a key to potty training success. But you can't just let them be hydrated and leave it at that. Potty training gives you a chance to be a student of your child. Learn which behaviors they exhibit before they need to relieve themselves. Study your child. It might sound stressful, but you can easily make it fun!

Being this focused does mean some sacrifice for you, though. Just think of it as stepping back into your grandma's or great-grandma's day and parenting the way they may have. You need to have focused attention on what needs to be done.

That means:

- No texting
- No phone calls
- No errands
- No distracting work

It means good, old-fashioned attentiveness to the needs of your child. Though it may sound like a burden at first, think about the impact some focused time on your child can have on your relationship, too! Your child might actually be more excited to just spend a day with Mommy or Daddy than they are about big-girl or big-boy undies.

Do I Need to Lock Myself at Home for a Week?

No way. Please don't. I know I would be a crazy person if I didn't leave the house at least once a day, and so would my children! I neither expect nor encourage you to stay trapped in your bathroom with your toddler for days on end. That's a formula to make anyone go crazy and act irrationally.

I highly suggest that you set aside at least one full day, and ideally two to three consecutive days, to focus on potty training. The efforts you put in now will pay off later. The first stage will be dedicated to studying your child and taking them to the toilet every time they start going. You'll be teaching them to move from "I went" to "I'm going." Then the second stage is transitioning from "I'm going" to "I need to go." The third stage is moving from "I need to go" to "I'm taking myself to the potty, because I need to go." And the final stage is post–dedicated potty training time. You want them to move to the ability to be able to recognize when a younger sibling or child needs to go.

Life happens and you may need to respond to an emergency, but don't plan for that. Plan to have your phone on silent, to take a day off of work, to simply focus on getting that pee and poo in the potty. Chapter 11: Special Circumstances (page 125) has tips for parents who can't spend a full first day (or two or three) potty training. The more focused attention you put in up front, the greater the long-term rewards.

Your days will look like the flowchart on the facing page.

I would encourage short trips out of the house after your child has at least 50 percent success of getting it in the potty at home, after the first day, or whenever you feel like you're going a bit stir crazy. Fresh air does wonders for a burdened heart.

Though I don't encourage running errands on the first day, please do take some quick breathers and get some fresh air. Once you've had a pee-ing success, wipe your child and be on your way outside for a five-minute adventure to watch ants crawling around, or to count blades of grass. Nothing overly planned. Nothing lasting more than five to ten minutes. Then go back inside, get them back into their potty training gear, and keep observing.

THE POTTY TRAINING CYCLE

PEE/POO SIGN (OR ACCIDENT)

Start again

Notice (verbally)

Get into potty
training gear

Respond
(verbally and physically)

Come back inside

Get it in the potty

Take a quick breather
outside (after you
have about 50 percent
success in the potty
at home)

Respond
(with your motivator of
choice)

- Check the mail
- Take the dog out to poop
- Watch ants
- Count blades of grass
- Talk about what the clouds look like (but remember to keep an eye on your child's peeing!)

- Clean out the car
- Walk down the street (not in a stroller)
- Wash a few windows
- Water a few plants with a watering can (Try not to get your child wet so that you can tell with assurance if they have an accident.)

What Do I Do When I'm at Home?

Hydrate and observe. That's the name of the game. Provide some form of hydration, through both drink and food. Anything from water to watered-down juice to soup broth is acceptable. Then you watch. You can switch between salty and sweet foods so that your child's appetite is whetted for a hydrating drink. Then as soon as your child starts to go, you notice and you respond.

Notice and respond. Over and over and over again. Notice and respond. Notice and respond. It's that simple; that is the main potty training process of this whole book. Notice what's going on and respond to it.

If your child is starting to squirm, say, "It looks like you're squirming" (that's the noticing part), and then respond to it with, "Go put your pee pee in the potty." Then walk them over to the toilet or pick them up and move them. It's your decision as to how you get them to the potty or toilet; just get them there.

Notice: "It looks like you're grabbing yourself."
Respond: "It's time to put that poo poo in the potty."

Notice: "You're doing a pee pee dance."
Respond: "Go run to the bathroom and sit on the toilet!"

How Do I Know That My Child Needs to Go?

You will need to start observing your child and paying attention to what is happening as they are going—and even more importantly, *just before* they are going. Let's review some common indicators that your child needs to poop or pee.

INDICATORS OF THE NEED TO POOP:

- Hiding to find privacy; common places are behind the couch, behind a curtain, behind a door, or in a solitary room or closet
- Grimacing or making a "poop face"
- Grunting
- Squatting
- Grabbing the back of a diaper or underwear

INDICATORS OF THE NEED TO PEE:

- Doing a "pee pee dance," usually indicated by crossing legs and some sort of bouncing around
- Grabbing groin area
- Crossing legs at the crotch
- Fidgeting
- Shifting weight while seated, like moving from one side of the chair to the other

Be prepared. This step takes the longest to master for most parents. It can take anywhere from three hours to a few days, and for certain special-needs parents it may take over two weeks. The longer it takes, the more breaks for yourself you need to build into the schedule.

STEP 4

KEEP A ROUTINE

Generally speaking, I'm not a fan of potty timers and potty watches, except in specialized situations. That said, keeping a schedule is *very* helpful in expediting potty training at home. Schedules also help your child transition well to pottying success at preschool or in other environments.

The general rule for when to take your child to the potty is: **Take them before putting them in or when taking them out of something.** This means offering them the chance to go before getting into a car seat, when getting out of a high chair, before they get into bed, and upon waking when they get out of bed.

It's Not Just a Matter of Timing

Yes, there are some logistics in potty training, but mostly it's an art. There are ebbs and flows. If your child had a late night the evening before, things might be tougher the next day. If you solely rely on a timer to take them, you miss actually figuring out when their body is telling them to go. They are being trained to go by the sound of the alarm, instead of by the sensation of a full bladder. Technically, you are making a sound association instead of a physical association. Unfortunately, when the sound is taken away, children often have no other association to encourage them to use the potty, and therefore regress. The method of a timer or alarm is actually closer to the method I suggest for babies practicing elimination communication than it is to potty training.

When you are starting to potty train, it's more effective to rely on when your child actually needs to go, rather than a timer. Again, remember that general rule above: Take your child to the potty before putting them *in* or when taking them *out of* something.

When Should I Take My Child to the Potty?

How does that general rule actually play out? Here's a sample schedule of the first day of potty training. It can be minimized after you get a sense of when your child actually needs to go. For example, on day three you might not need to take your child before and after a snack because you learned they only go after . . . but you won't know that on day one. This schedule is to help you learn your child's natural routine. Use the below as a reference guide to create your family's pottying schedule.

FOR DAYTIME: WHEN TO TAKE YOUR CHILD TO THE POTTY

- Ideally within 5 to 10 minutes of waking up; if they're still half asleep that early, just take within 20 minutes of waking
- Before breakfast
- After breakfast
- Upon arriving at an activity (such as preschool)
- Before snack time
- After snack time
- Before lunch
- After lunch
- Before nap
- After nap
- Before snack
- After snack
- Before dinner
- After dinner
- Before getting ready for bed (meaning before bath, jammies, or reading a book)
- Directly before getting into bed
- Whenever they show you they need to go
- Whenever they've gone only a drop or two, but you know they need to go more
- Anytime you're already going, take them with you

Does more than 16 times in one day sound like too many? Think about the methods that suggest taking your child every 10 to 15 minutes. Assuming they're awake for 12 hours and take a two-hour nap, that's 10 hours of awake time. There are four 15-minute periods in each hour and six 10-minute periods per hour, so that's 40 to 60 bathroom trips during awake hours!

FOR NIGHTTIME: WHEN TO TAKE YOUR CHILD TO THE POTTY

Take your child to the bathroom at these added times if they are not staying dry throughout the night.

- One to two hours after falling asleep. If they "go to bed" at 6:30 p.m., but don't fall asleep until 7:00 p.m., take them between 8:00 p.m. and 9:00 p.m.
- One to two hours before waking up. If they wake up at 6:00 a.m., then take them between 4:00 a.m. and 5:00 a.m. For this waking, you have the liberty to move it earlier so that your little one's sleep habits aren't affected as much. We don't want them waking for the day at 4:00 a.m.!

For additional details about nap time and nighttime potty training, see Chapter 7: Nighttime and Napping (page 94).

The Power Your Preschool Has over Pottying

Since preschools are the ones who can put your child back in diapers at the drop of the hat, when push comes to shove, they generally have the "ultimate" say over whether your child wears diapers at preschool. You probably agreed to this when you signed your child's preschool admittance contract.

Yes, you can argue and call meetings and lay down the law with them, but generally speaking, this isn't a hill to die on. They are providing multiple other things to your child, like food, stimulus, safety, cleanliness, and education. They have multiple other children to care for as well. Your child's potty training is not their number one priority, nor should it be.

We don't want to become an enemy to those who are trying their best to love and teach our children. We want to respect them, and honor the authority that we have given them in our children's and family's lives.

In order to help your child and your preschool staff make the transition from home to preschool, try your best to mirror their pottying schedule for your child. We will go over this in more detail in Chapter 9: Family and Other Caregivers (page 108).

How Do I Get My Child to Stay on the Toilet?

It's not a matter of sitting on the toilet for 20 minutes at a time, or even all day. Please don't do that! By forcing your child to sit on the potty or toilet when they don't need to go, you are actually creating an association in their little brain that they are potty training just to please you. That's not the intent at all. You don't want them to sit on the potty to please you. We want their mind and body to start having the association that "when I feel like I need to go pee pee or poo poo, I run to the bathroom and can put it there and then leave."

If your child is not actively peeing or pooping after one to two minutes, or at least earnestly trying to, have them leave the toilet. They can try again in a few minutes if they need to, but don't just have them sit there. Even if they sit there willingly using electronics or reading a book, unless they are actually pottying, they can do those things elsewhere. They don't need to learn that the only time Mommy will read them a book is when they're on the potty. Go grab a book and sit on the couch or on the floor, and read to them.

For kids who sit for less than 30 seconds, here are some tactics to get them to stay on the potty or toilet long enough to even feel the sensation of needing to go:

- Use the actual toilet instead of a mini potty, as it's farther from the floor and children are less likely to get down from it and run off.
- Face them backward; for some kids, especially those with smaller bottoms, they feel much more secure placed backward and are less likely

to pop off. They can also watch the pee or poo fall in, which is fun for some kids.

■ Give them something to do while on the potty, but nothing too distracting. Good options are a book with flaps in it or jelly stickers to use on the inside of the lid while facing backward.

Encourage your child to focus on pottying while on the toilet by saying something like the following:

■ "Once you get your poo/pee in the potty you can go and _____."

■ "Since you're already on the potty, might as well put the poo/pee in it!"

■ "Try to relax your stomach muscles and just let it fall out."

■ For kids who are scared of pooping, personifying the poop can help alleviate their fears. You can do that by "naming" the poop and then asking it to come out. This isn't your standard potty training method, but for kids who are scared because of past constipation issues, it can be a game changer. "Let Mr. Poo Poo come out and go for a swim in the water."

■ "What a big boy/girl you are sitting on there going potty!"

Remember, you don't want to be overbearing and pushy. You want to focus on being encouraging.

STEP 5
REACT TO THEIR BEHAVIOR

Typically, this stage involves offering praise and rewards. People often suggest giving your child a sticker or a small piece of candy. However, I think that we need to consider all the options and weigh them against the choices we make as a family, the values we each have, and the preferences we want to use in order to motivate our children.

Choosing how to react to their successes can be a crucial part of your overall parenting strategy. Is it worth a huge debate to decide? By all means, no. But if you have a bit of time to mull it over, talk with your co-parent about how you think it is best to motivate your child. M&M's are not the only option.

QUESTIONS TO CONSIDER:

- Do we want to offer them praise for good behavior?
- Do we want them to expect good behavior of themselves and be rewarded only when something is out of the range of normal?
- Do we praise effort?
- Do we praise success?
- Do we praise materialistically?
- Do we praise verbally?

If you choose to praise verbally, you'll want to think about what you're going to say. Don't worry; I'll give you some ideas at the end of this section.

There are numerous theories that describe motivation: the theory of motivation, drive theories, the arousal theory of motivation, and others. Essentially, what we care about is whether our children are driven by internal or external motivators: extrinsic or intrinsic motivation. You will learn more about each in Chapter 5: Your Child, Your Choice (page 72).

The basic difference lies in whether you plan to motivate your child internally or externally. Are they motivated from within, or are there factors outside of themselves that are motivating them to take a certain action?

For the sake of potty training, motivation often falls into two categories:

- Extrinsic: Do you give rewards and praise?
- Intrinsic: Do you set an expectation and teach them to reach that new "normal" of their own initiative?

Through both extrinsic and intrinsic motivation, you can teach children the rails of the direction you want them to follow. You can teach them that it's a new norm to be followed, or you can teach them that they will be rewarded for their positive behavior. It's your choice, and you can always swap later if the one you choose now isn't working for you.

How to Encourage Your Child

If you're looking for ways to encourage your child along the journey, taking a moment to consider their "love language" could open up a whole new world of possibilities. With over 11 million copies sold, *The 5 Love Languages* by Gary Chapman shows methods of encouragement that have been used worldwide. The book provides options for how to encourage your child and can easily be applied to potty training. They can be game changers for how your children perceive you and how well cared for by you they feel.

1. WORDS OF AFFIRMATION: This love language uses words to affirm other people.
    For this child, hearing that you are proud of them, that you love them, and that you think they're doing a wonderful job can be a huge motivating factor for them.

2. ACTS OF SERVICE: For these people, actions speak louder than words.
    This child might not care that you sang a song when they peed, but their little heart might feel very full if you do something as simple as getting a new roll of toilet paper, cleaning up a mess off the floor, grabbing clean clothes for them, or bringing their favorite book to the potty for them.

3. RECEIVING GIFTS: For some people, what makes them feel most loved is to receive a gift.
    This is the child for whom the well-thought-out sticker chart or the prize basket is very motivating. But don't just buy "stuff"; buy something with *this* specific child in mind, and tell them why you picked out that special gift for them.

4. QUALITY TIME: This love language is all about giving the other person your undivided attention.

Do something together. Listen to your child's newest story, song, or joke. Play Legos. Have a quality interaction. Maybe even get a sitter for other children so that you can focus on just this child.

5. PHYSICAL TOUCH: To this person, nothing speaks more deeply than appropriate touch.

    Think in terms of hugs, cuddles, and time spent reading while sitting on your lap or leaning against you. It could even be something as simple as holding hands.

If you give a child who is encouraged by words a sticker as a reward, they are less likely to feel loved and encouraged. Take a minute to think about how your child responds to each of these love languages and choose a method or two that will be motivating for them. If you're not sure which to choose, Chapman's book is a worthwhile read.

Phrases of Praise

While your child is making progress, you may choose to encourage them along the way through verbal praise. If you choose to do so, here are some sample phrases of encouragement with which to praise your child. Think about your child. Some kids will respond and feel encouraged if you call them a big kid. Others will cry at the loss of not being a baby anymore. Just think about who your child is before trying to encourage them.

The following are listed in a progressive order:

- **"You can do it!"** Before starting potty training, encourage your child. First, believe it yourself; then you will contagiously have them believing they can do it, too! As my mom always says, "It's the power of positive thinking!"
- **"You've giving such good effort!"** This is a perfect phrase for a little one who is trying oh-so hard, but isn't quite making it in the toilet. They sure are giving a lot of effort, but they aren't actually doing a "good job" yet.
- **"You're making progress!"** The child who is giving great effort and is having a reasonable amount of success often needs to be

encouraged in the progress that they have already made. You can
remind them of the "silly" times they peed on the floor in the kitchen,
or when they used diapers "like a baby."

- **"You're doing such a great job!"** This is a wonderful phrase for children who are near completion, as it suggests that they have already
  mastered the art of whatever they're doing.
- **"If you need me, just ask! I'm here for you."** Use this phrase for
  a child who is nearly pottying on their own. This is the child whom
  you want to encourage to do every step independently, but who can't
  physically do them all yet. You want to encourage autonomy while
  letting them know you'll support them along the way. Stay close by.
- **"You're doing it!"** This reminds me of the movie *Hook*, where the
  adult version of Peter Pan is trying to learn to use his imagination to
  play with the Lost Boys. One starts saying it and the others chime in,
  saying, "You're doing it, Peter!" There's a whole group encouraging
  the same behavior. Let others know to help encourage your child with
  potty training success. It's not pressure at this point. It's sheer recog-
  nition of a job well done. You want that community of people cheering
  on your child, saying, "You're doing it, [your child's name]!"

This chapter conveys the bulk of the potty training process. You are
in the thick of it when you are in this stage. Be encouraged that this
is the hardest and most time-consuming part. Picture the long-term
vision: heading over to a friend's house and continuing an actual conversation after your child says, "I have to potty." Your child heads to the
bathroom on their own, completing each step independently, from A
to Z. It's not instantaneous, but it will happen. The foundation you lay
now instills good habits that will easily be mimicked in other areas of
your child's life as well.

A NOTE FOR SPECIAL-NEEDS PARENTS

If the reality for you is that your child may never be capable of completing all the steps independently, be encouraged that I am cheering you on regardless! I will celebrate any of the learning that happens along this journey. My favorite part of my job is hearing from parents who have been told that their child isn't capable of X, Y, or Z, who then tell me of all the progress that their child actually made, despite the naysayers. I celebrate the incremental successes with you!

FIVE

Your Child,
Your Choice

MAKING THE PLAN YOUR OWN

Now, how do we cram your unique child into this one-size-fits-all plan? We don't. We adjust the plan to fit your family, your lifestyle, and your child. We'll modify the plan around what I call the "big rocks." That means we'll figure out the most important factors, and then develop a plan around what's most important to your family. We'll keep the basic structure of the plan outlined in chapter 4 intact, but tweak it a bit to mold to the needs and preferences of your family.

What to Wear

There are various factors that go into making the decision of what to dress your child in for potty training:

- Where do you live?
- What's the weather?
- What season are you potty training in?
- Indoors or outside?
- Do you feel comfortable with your child naked outside in this digital- photo-taking world?
- What does your co-parent feel comfortable with?

You get to decide the clothes that your child wears during potty training. I would *highly* recommend making this decision *with* your co-parent ahead of time. The last thing you want is your co-parent to come home angry when they find their child running around the house naked. I don't encourage you to ever let a naked toddler out of your sight! Don't feel like you are committing to this decision for the long haul. I highly suggest updating this plan as you progress so you don't end up with a potty trained toddler who refuses to wear underwear.

GARMENT TRAINING OPTIONS:

- Naked (totally naked):
  - **If you have not practiced "elimination communication," this step is HIGHLY recommended. The learning curve is great for recognizing your child's signs that they need to pee or poo. Your child being naked will expedite your learning process.** That being said, you could choose from the other options, as well, but it will be slower and you will have more misses.
  - "Naked" just means being able to see your child's private parts when they go. This can include options such as leg warmers.

- Naked from waist down (shirt on top half):
  - See notes above, but consider that you won't be fully able to see what's going on when the pee/poo arrives if you choose a shirt that's as long as a short dress.
  - Feel free to pair with some "naked" options as well, such as leg warmers or BabyLegs.
- Commando (pants/skirt/shorts, but no underwear or diaper): This could include a shirt or not, your choice. This also includes crotchless pants.
- Sumo style (cloth diaper with prefold diaper belt): Your child is covered, and you have easy access to take off their backup (the cloth diaper). Because of the thickness of the cloth, this often causes a delay in noticing that they have wet or soiled themselves.
- Just undies: This means just having your child wear underwear or training undies. I don't recommend potty training in Pull-Ups.
- Regular clothes: This includes outer garment (such as pants/dress/shorts) and an undergarment—in this case, underwear or training undies.

As a general rule, plan to add a garment before leaving the house. Some examples include the following:

- You were naked training and now you're having your child commando (you added a dress or pants/shorts)
- You were training commando in the house in a skirt and now you're adding shorts under the skirt
- You were training commando in the house in pants and now you're adding undies under the pants

That's it. Decide your starting garments for potty training and take it from there! Don't forget to talk to your co-parent about it as well.

EXTRA TRICKS AND TIPS

Normalize, Normalize, Normalize

I cannot stress this enough. The more "normal" that a child views using the potty, the more likely they are to assimilate to using it without complaint. Try to make it like a chair that you sit on while eating dinner or a couch that you sit on while watching TV. It is just a place where you sit when you're peeing or pooping. Make it normal. Make the other places for peeing or pooing abnormal.

The old normal was peeing and pooping while sitting eating dinner. The old normal was peeing and pooping while watching TV. The "new normal" is peeing and pooping on the potty. Every. Single. Time.

You need them to believe they can do it. They need to know that you want the new normal to be true. Every. Single. Time. In order for that to happen, *you* need to believe it, too. You need to care that it happens. Every. Single. Time. You need to exemplify that it is normal.

How Do You Make Pottying "Normal" to a Child?

MAKE A POTTY ACCESSIBLE

- Don't put a potty seat in Mommy and Daddy's room unless you want your child to use it in there without asking you every time.
- If they can't reach the toilet without a stool, provide a stool.
- Put a potty within eyesight of a child when they are able to use it. I don't recommend strapping a diapered child into a high chair and then putting a potty in the kitchen hoping they'll put the pieces together. Even if they do, there's not much they can do about it instantaneously. But putting a potty on the floor in the kitchen when a child is walking around with just stretchy pants on . . . that's helpful!

HAVE A "POTTY PARTY"

- We're not talking streamers and Pin the Tail on the Donkey. What I mean is that when you can incorporate others whom you trust to be part of the pottying process, that is nearly always a win. I suggest having older siblings exemplify how to use the potty and how to wash up afterward. Maybe have a neighbor kid come over and help show your child. Obviously, use your discretion, but having an older child can do wonders to normalize the whole process, especially if your younger child looks up to that older one.
- As a note of caution, be wary of making your child feel comfortable around all strangers while pottying. I teach elimination communication classes for parents of infants ages 0 to 18 months and have often been asked by students if they can watch as I potty my babies. Though I earnestly want my students to learn, I just don't feel comfortable with my children feeling watched when they potty. You're the parent, and you get to decide what you're comfortable with.

READ POTTYING BOOKS TO YOUR CHILD

- Don't feel like you have to buy every potty training board book on the market. Just grab a few good ones.
- You can tell your children stories about characters they like and include that so-and-so had to stop after lunch to take a potty trip and then continue the story. Just make it a fact in the story and move on.

HAVE YOUR CHILD GO WHEN YOU GO

- Whenever you need to go to the bathroom (assuming you have a mini potty so your child can go at the same time), take your child with you. This will help them learn that there are "normal" times to use the potty, such as upon waking or after a meal.

HAVE AN "I DID IT" UNDIES PHOTO SHOOT

■ A few quick snaps of the phone camera to commemorate the occasion can help instill in your child a sense of "I did it!" as a past-tense action. This will help them learn that potty training is a thing of the past and dry undies are a new normal for them, and you!

FAQ

I don't feel comfortable with naked training. Do I have to do that?

No, not at all. As stated before, it almost always expedites the potty training process, but you don't have to. Your child can wear anything from commando (pants/dress without undies), to undies, to training undies, to a sumo-style cloth diaper, to BabyLegs under a dress, to pants and undies. The rule of thumb to keep in mind is this: The closer you are to the source of the pee or poo, the quicker you'll be able to react when they go. The faster you react, the better your child will be at making the connection between feeling the need to go and actually releasing.

I'm germaphobic and don't want to use public restrooms. Can I modify this plan so that I don't have to?

Absolutely. Travel potties will be your best friend. I have already suggested some in Chapter 3: Are You Ready? (page 30). If you have a larger vehicle, like a van or SUV, you can actually have your child potty in your car. You might want to put down a piddle pad, a towel, or a tarp before setting up the potty, because cleaning vehicle carpet can be a bother. Most travel potties also have some sort of disposable liner or bag as well. Just set up that travel potty and have your child go before and after heading somewhere in the car, and you'll be golden.

Should I teach my boy to go sitting down or standing up?

Most potty training–age boys aren't quite tall enough to stand up and get their penis over the ledge of a public restroom's toilet or the side of a urinal. For the sake of germs and cleanup, it's often simpler to just teach them to sit down backward (facing the tank) on the toilet. Of course, this often requires you to pick them up. If you have a baby in arms to take with you to a public restroom, think this situation through ahead of time. Baby carriers are a perfect solution.

I have children close in age or we had a multiple birth. Should I potty train them all at the same time? Which one should I potty train first?

Generally, I suggest that you start potty training the less strong-willed child first. Then, after they start at least somewhat understanding and following suit, take the diapers off the other child as well. I know many suggest getting the "leader" on board, but I've learned that the leader will often attempt a mutiny, where a more compliant child is more likely to adapt. The stronger-willed child will often voluntarily check in on the action because they want to catch up on whatever new thing is going on.

How do you handle potty training when your child is being disciplined?

Often, being sent to time-out is enough of an emotional and physical trigger that a child legitimately needs to potty. Let them go to the potty once. You could choose to let them go in the bathroom or bring a potty to them. But, whatever you do, don't let them sit on the potty and play. They need to be actively peeing or pooing; otherwise they can finish their time-out. It's not as though time-outs are 20 minutes long. If they go during time-out, don't give them any fun potty books. They are either in play mode or in time-out—not both.

Ask a Parent

How did you adapt the potty training plan for your own personal needs?

"I bought a book bag and it's how I carry my little one's potty seat, Lysol spray, Lysol wipes, hand sanitizer, and a change of clothes. Plus, rewards are in the front pocket." —LINDA

"When I felt I understood her well enough, and that she understood me well enough, I started to take steps to build interest in my daughter for the potty beyond her own personal hatred of diapers. We bought dolls, books, talked about the potty and we made the potty a member of our family for a month to artificially instill an interest in it. My husband and I would even celebrate when either of us went potty and let my daughter cheer *us* on, to see if we could really build that excitement. Once the excitement was there, combined with her ability to follow instructions and desire to be diaper free, I knew we were going to be successful, despite the hundreds of people (including my own mother!) who said she was too young." —GERALDINE

SIX

Pooping and Peeing

Welcome to the poop-and-pee chapter. You've made it to the depths of parenting! Let's get to it. Often people choose to potty train in "levels"; maybe pee before poo or poo before pee. As a general rule, here is the order that most children gain bowel and bladder control:

- Nighttime poop control
- Daytime poop control
- Daytime pee control
- Nighttime pee control

It's helpful to go in this order if you are going from fully diapered to potty training quite young. Otherwise, if your child is 18 months of age or above, I recommend potty training for both poop and pee at the same time. We all know that potty training isn't a one-size-fits-all process, but here are my suggestions:

1. If at all possible, potty train for both poop and pee at the same time (for 18+ months)

2. Second choice would be to potty train for poop first and then pee

3. Third choice would be to potty train for pee and later poop (not recommended—why would you want poopy diapers more than pee diapers?)

There are a variety of opinions regarding how long it takes a child to potty train for pee after they have already been trained to poop in the toilet, or vice versa. It can be anywhere from a few days to a month or two. This is why I highly suggest training for both at the same time. This can often be best achieved by potty training naked, since many children will wait until they get their diaper back and then poop. You can also train for both at the same time by devoting a few days in a row to potty training. If you are fully committed one day and then pop them back into a diaper for preschool the next day, and then take off the diaper the day after that, it's very likely that your child will adjust their bowel habits to pooping only when they have a diaper on. This is likely to produce a child who is in a habit of pooping at preschool in a diaper. If your child has been successful at home diaper free and you ask your preschool to stop using a diaper as well, you may end up with a child with preschool poop accidents. Taking those few days in a row and dedicating your time to potty training can help teach your child that poop and pee go in the toilet, around the clock, from day one.

NORMAL PEE AND POOP

We live in an age where we typically don't forage for greens that fill our plates or delight in seasonal, fresh, organic produce that was picked that day. If you're a meat eater, we tend to include far more meat in our diets than we actually need. The amount of fiber we get is minimal in comparison to our ancestors, and thus we need to be more sensitive to our tendency to become constipated. Even if you don't think your child is constipated, this section is worth a quick skim. You may be surprised at what constipation actually is.

Is My Child Constipated?

In case you were wondering, there actually is a very systematic way of figuring out whether your child's poop is normal, thanks to the work of Dr. Stephen Lewis and Dr. Ken Heaton at the University Department of Medicine at Bristol Royal Infirmary in England. The Bristol Stool Scale is a great reference guide to figure out if your child (or you!) has constipation or diarrhea.

According to the Bristol Stool Scale, the seven types of stool are:

- Type 1: Separate hard lumps, like nuts (hard to pass); also known as *goat faeces*
- Type 2: Sausage shaped but lumpy
- Type 3: Like a sausage but with cracks on its surface
- Type 4: Like a sausage or snake, smooth and soft
- Type 5: Soft blobs with clearcut edges (passed easily)
- Type 6: Fluffy pieces with ragged edges, a mushy stool
- Type 7: Watery, no solid pieces, entirely liquid

Types 1 and 2 indicate constipation, 3 and 4 are the ideal stools (especially the latter) as they are easy to defecate while not containing excess liquid, and 5, 6, and 7 tend toward diarrhea. According to the initial study in "The Bristol Scale" by M. Mínguez Pérez and A. Benages Martínez, types 1 and 2 stools were more prevalent in females, while types 5 and 6 stools were more prevalent in males; furthermore, 80 percent of subjects who reported rectal tenesmus (urgency to defecate) had type 7.

BRISTOL STOOL CHART

Type 1	
Type 2	
Type 3	
Type 4	
Type 5	
Type 6	
Type 7	

WHAT YOUR CHILD IS FEELING RIGHT NOW

Running away from the toilet. Crying. Screaming. Saying, "I'm scared." These can all be common symptoms that go along with a child learning to poop in the potty, especially if they are constipated. If a child needs to strain in order to poop, it can be anything from uncomfortable, to painful, to semitraumatic (seeing blood in the toilet).

For the average child who is just used to the feel of poop pressed up against their skin, it feels odd at minimum and scary at most. For some children it's a surprise, like if someone all of a sudden blew in your face. You'd react. You'd be surprised. You might be a little angry that they did it. Understand and be sympathetic to the fact that it's a new sensation and might be a bit of a transition. Remember that new doesn't mean bad. Just because they are surprised doesn't mean they need a diaper back.

WHAT DO I DO IF MY CHILD IS CONSTIPATED?

Constipation can often be cured naturally, but not always. If natural remedies are not curing your child's constipation, please do seek the medical advice of a physician.

Natural Remedies:

- **Drink Water:** For children ages 1 to 3, the Dietary Reference Intakes (DRI) for water, including food, beverages, and drinking water, is 44 ounces per day.
- **Exercise:** Moving helps to move that poop through your child's system. Sitting at preschool, watching a movie, or even sitting on the toilet for extended periods of time can be very counterproductive. If you're trying to get your child to poop, get them moving. Then when they do stop moving, it most often will be a very clear sign that they need to pee or poo.
- **Fiber-Rich Foods:** Fiber-rich foods are an excellent remedy to fight your child's constipation. I will go into depth on this in How Much Fiber Does a Child Need? on page 89.
- **Probiotics:** Though often recommended, probiotics need to be used prudently. According to a study conducted by the Department of Pediatrics, Ospedale Civile Maggiore at the University of Verona, Italy, constipated children actually showed a significant increase in the amount of clostridia and bifidobacteria in their feces, as compared with healthy children. Please consult your physician before administering probiotics as a treatment for constipation.

Be wary that chronic constipation in children can actually be caused by a variety of underlying medical conditions. According to Stephen M. Borowitz, MD, at the University of Virginia School of Medicine, the range of reasons for diagnosis of childhood constipation can be extensive.

What Does Healthy Urine Look Like?

According to the United States National Library of Medicine, urine is typically straw yellow in color. Characteristics of abnormal urine include being cloudy, dark, or blood colored. Colors that are abnormal may be caused by various factors, including foods, infection, disease, and medicines. Urine may also be affected by vitamins and artificial coloring in your foods or beverages.

HERE'S A LOOK AT THE "RAINBOW" OF URINE TYPES:

Note: This is not medical advice, and any concerns should to brought up to your physician.

Clear: Water-like consistency. This means your child is drinking too much water and ought to cut back.

Milky or Cloudy: Your child may have a urinary tract infection (UTI). There may also be a bad smell to the urine if they have a UTI. Go to a physician to have them tested. Milky or cloudy urine "may also be caused by bacteria, crystals, fat, white or red blood cells, or mucus in the urine," according to the United States National Library of Medicine.

Pink or Red: This can be caused by eating beets, blackberries, or artificial food dye; vaginal bleeding; and a host of other more severe ailments.

Orange or Dark Yellow: These colors come from medicines (such as some used to treat a UTI), orange Gatorade, laxatives, or vitamins and minerals, such as B complex vitamins or carotene.

Straw-like Yellow: This is ideal. Keep it up! Your child is well hydrated, but not overdoing the water.

Green or Blue: Urine in these colors comes from artificial coloring, medicines, UTIs, or bilirubin.

Dark Brown (but Clear): This can be an indication of a liver disorder.

THE "RAINBOW" OF URINE TYPES

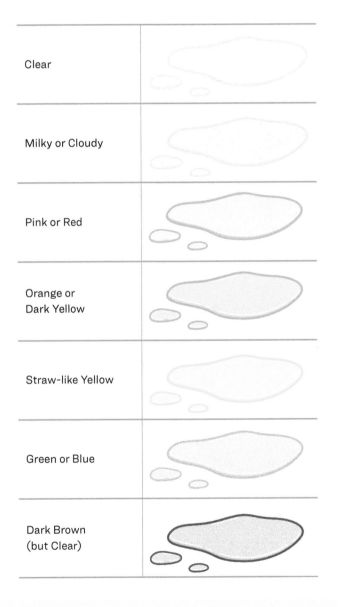

Clear	
Milky or Cloudy	
Pink or Red	
Orange or Dark Yellow	
Straw-like Yellow	
Green or Blue	
Dark Brown (but Clear)	

Practicing with Your Child

Over a sink or bowl filled with water, take a gumball-sized ball of Play-Doh and push it through your fingers so that it drops into the water. Explain to your child that it is just like poop falling from their bottom into the toilet. It may make a noise, it may splash, but that's how it comes out and it's all going to be okay.

FAQ

How do I teach my child how to wipe?

First of all, tell your child *why* they are wiping. They're learning to wipe so that they don't get sick from the germs, are not stinky, stay clean, and don't get itchy.

For Poop:

- Make sure they know that they are trying to wipe off all of the poop.
- Teach your child to pull off a specific amount of toilet paper.

For Girls:

- Wipe from front to back (from vagina to anus) to avoid urinary tract infections, commonly called UTIs.
- Sometimes using the word *blotting* makes more sense to a girl instead of "wiping" themselves.

My child hides to poop. Does that mean they're ready to start potty training or that they need more time to learn not to be embarrassed about their poop?

If a child is physically removing themselves from a situation with others to seek out privacy to pee and poo, wouldn't this be the perfect time to teach them where it goes? It's just the next step in the process. If they

HOW MUCH FIBER DOES A CHILD NEED?

In accordance with the Dietary Reference Intakes published by the National Institutes of Health, the recommended fiber intake for a child of one to three years old is 19 grams per day. Jennifer Zils of the website Kids Eat Vegetables makes it her goal to help parents navigate proper nutrition for their children. She has kindly provided us with a list of kid-friendly, fiber-rich foods, with their fiber counts. Nutritional information is based on the United States Department of Agriculture Agricultural Research Service's Food Composition Database.

Top Kid-Friendly, Fiber-Rich Foods

- Acorn squash, baked: 1 cup, cubed = 9.0 grams (g)
- Apple with skin: 1 cup quartered = 3.0g, small-sized = 3.6g
- Avocado, puréed: ½ cup = 7.8g
- Banana: 1 cup, sliced = 3.9g, 1 small = 2.6g
- Black beans, canned: ½ cup = 8.3g
- Broccoli, boiled: 1 cup, chopped = 2.6g
- Blueberries: 1 cup = 3.6g
- Chia seeds: 1 ounce = 9.8g
- Fig, dried: 2 pieces = 5.0g
- Oatmeal: 1 packet (41g) = 4g
- Pear with skin: 1 cup, sliced = 4.3g, 1 small = 4.6g
- Popcorn, popped: 1 cup = 1.1g
- Raspberries: 1 cup = 8.0g
- Strawberries: 1 cup, sliced = 3.3g
- Sweet potatoes, boiled without skin: 1 cup, mashed = 8.2g
- 100 percent whole-grain bread: 2 slices = 4.6g
- Whole-grain pasta: 1 cup elbow pasta = 12.3g

were an animal and left the group to go poop, it would be socially acceptable for them to hide it in a bush or a hole somewhere.

Let's give our children the dignity of teaching them where it is socially acceptable to put that pee and poo. Even if you as the parent aren't ready to get rid of diapers right away, please still do them the favor of teaching them where the pee and poo go. If you choose not to potty train yet, then it is still a good time to teach them how to dispose of used diapers. For example, dump poop in the toilet, then wrap the diaper up on itself and toss in the trash, laundry basket, or diaper pail.

As far as embarrassment goes, most kids aren't embarrassed about pooping until someone points out that they're doing it in their diaper, when other similarly aged kids are using the potty. That seems to be the main source of embarrassment. Giving a child more time to figure it out on their own doesn't give them the resources they need to understand what poop is and where it should go. Here's your perfect chance to teach them!

My child is already peeing in the toilet. How do I teach them to poop in the toilet, too?

Generally speaking, if this issue is happening, I'm guessing that your child is wearing diapers or Pull-Ups part-time. Is that true? A lot of the time children will store up their poop until they're handed a Pull-Up or a diaper is put back on. Whenever that moment is, it's time break the habit. Be okay with a few messes for the sake of no more poopy diapers. When you get rid of the diapers this time, make it for real.

I highly recommend around-the-clock training for a child who is continuing to poop while in bed during a nap or at night. Be forewarned, though, that a manipulative child who is used to pooping right after being given a diaper or Pull-Up at nap time or nighttime isn't going to be very happy when you take it away. There may be tears. There will probably be screaming and fits. Keep in mind that they will still probably need to poop. That means you still need to watch them like a hawk, especially if they are "almost" asleep.

WHAT IF YOUR CHILD'S POOP SMELLS STRANGE?

Generally speaking, poop smells unpleasant, but it is a familiar unpleasant smell. According to the United States National Library of Medicine, "Stools that have an extremely bad, abnormal odor may be due to certain medical conditions. Foul-smelling stools also have normal causes, such as diet changes."

My child is already pooping in the toilet. How do I teach them to pee in the toilet, too?

Boys and girls can be a bit different in this aspect of potty training. The anatomy of a boy just makes it easier for them to pee and to not worry about where it goes (if they are naked) because it doesn't affect them physically. As it is, a naked peeing boy often doesn't get wet, so what does it matter to him if he peed across the living room floor? For girls, they are often inconvenienced by the wetness running down their legs and want help cleaning up. That said, how to do you help teach them?

For a boy, putting him *in* undies to potty train for pee can often be the most effective way because it causes him to feel the wetness.

For a girl, having her in undies causes her to feel the wetness without causing a big mess. Whatever you've been trying with a girl (undies or no undies), just try the reverse.

If it has been an ongoing issue for a boy or girl (let's say past a week), you may want to monitor hydration and set a reminder for yourself to take them to the bathroom about 20 minutes after they drink a full cup.

If my child is having a lot of poop accidents, should I go back to diapers?

If at all possible, no. Here's a story from a parent who did go back to diapers after poop accidents, which illustrates why I do not recommend going back and forth between undies and diapers:

"We have been at this for four months. She has successfully peed more times than I can count. Pooped once. It's a nightmare for us. She has even stopped telling us if she's wet or pooped in her diaper. We end up going back and forth from undies to diapers. I feel like we are going to scar her, too. I think my daughter is faking and is just too lazy to stop her activities to go. Then when we say time to change her, she drags that out to the point of crawling to her changing room."

Is constipation "normal" for kids?

Unfortunately, pediatric constipation is a very common occurrence. But "common" doesn't make something "normal." Constipation should be viewed as an abnormal bowel habit, one to try to avoid.

Ask a Parent

How did you as parents with potty training experience handle poop training? (I don't recommend all of the below advice, but this worked for some parents.)

"We did continue the glycerin liquid suppositories [recommended by our doctor] every second or third day, which immediately did produce a bowel movement for her. It was not very traumatic as most people might think it would be. With lots of love and positive support she has been accident free for one month and will be returning to school with her brothers next month. I can't thank you enough for all of your help and resources." —LEONARD

"I wish I taught my daughter to poop in the potty first before taking her nappy off!" —ANDREA

"Increase fiber . . . and/or give SMALL amounts of prune juice (makes you go but also hurts tummy), or better (no pain) than the prune juice is apple juice. She won't have a choice but to let it out." —TAMARA

"I'd try three days of no underwear and no Pull-Ups. The Pull-Ups feel like a diaper. One or two accidents and he'll learn. My stubborn son just held it. I made sure he had apples and broccoli so he wouldn't get constipated. He keeps asking for a diaper. I told him that we had no more and no money to buy more. It took a couple of days. When he finally went, he said, 'That's not so bad.'" —DANA

SEVEN

Nighttime and Napping

HOW TO NIGHTTIME TRAIN

There are various ways you can nighttime train. I'll give you multiple options and then give you some pointers on how to choose the best method for your family. Before implementing any of these methods at night, I would suggest implementing a "double pee" before bedtime: Have your child go pee before their bedtime routine, and then once again directly before getting into bed.

Hydration

I don't recommend limiting water intake throughout the day as a preventive measure against bedwetting. Keep the hydration coming. However, if you're in potty training mode, you are probably being very diligent with hydration and you may need to go back to normal hydration before bedtime. Different children work in different ways, so feel free to try several methods from below to see what works best. I suggest starting from the top of this list and moving down if the technique isn't working.

Do the total opposite, allow liquids: I often recommend letting your child drink as much water as they'd like throughout the day and before bed. Often even a mention of restricting or forbidding water before bedtime makes your child want water, even though they really wouldn't care normally. It's not a matter of how much water they are getting; it's a matter of getting in the habit of drinking water before bed just because it's limited or forbidden. Some studies have shown bedwetting to be linked to constipation. If your child has a problem with bedwetting, it is likely that they also have a problem with constipation. They could be dealing with constipation for a myriad of reasons (see Chapter 6: Pooping and Peeing, page 80). Constipation can be aggravated by poor hydration. Thus, limiting hydration before bed could actually increase constipation and therefore bedwetting.

Reduce water before bed: This means that instead of a whole sippy cup, you should provide just a small (3 oz.) cup in the bathroom after bath time.

Restrict water before bed for one to two hours before bedtime: The idea here is that the less liquid there is in the bladder, the more likely your child will be able to hold the new urine until the morning.

If your child is used to pottying based on a timer or a schedule, I want your child to learn what it feels like to have a full bladder and to empty their bladder before going to bed. If you limit their water, you actually set them up to not feel like they need to void directly before getting into bed. That's more likely to send them to bed with urine in their system and have them feel like they need to go in the middle of the night. That said, using small cups can help so that they're not loading up so much on water. You don't want them to need to make more urine even after peeing before bed, which could lead to nighttime problems.

Different Approaches to Nighttime Training

1. WAKE AT SET TIMES (RECOMMENDED): The idea is that your child is able to actually urinate only at certain times during the night because of their sleep cycles, so you try to take them to use the toilet just before they will go through that next REM cycle. The catch is that toddlers' sleep cycles are anywhere from 50 to 90 minutes long, so there's not an exact science to it all. Generally speaking, the closer your child is to infant age, the shorter their sleep cycle.

   Wake at set times during the night, somewhere between 50 minutes and 90 minutes after your child falls asleep, and between 50 minutes and 90 minutes before they typically wake (or the 50 minutes to 90 minutes before that if you desire to avoid altering their wake-up time). Note that this is not upon putting to bed; instead, it's based upon the actual time of falling asleep.

2. WAKE AT SET TIMES AND THEN MOVE THOSE TIMES CLOSER TOGETHER (RECOMMENDED): This is for parents who know their child wakes up wet, but don't want to continually wake their child up twice a night in the long term. This is the fastest and most effective method of helping your child achieve nighttime dryness, assuming there are no underlying medical problems. This is a bit of a "choose your own adventure" method. The basic concept is that you are trying to merge two wake-up times into just one wake-up time. Then you slowly move that wake-up time later and later until the next time they need to pee is upon morning waking. Sleep is important, too!

3. WAIT FOR INDEPENDENT NIGHTTIME DRYNESS (NOT RECOMMENDED, EXCEPT IN INSTANCES OF PARENT MAINTENANCE MODE): This is a popular method that is endorsed on several diapering companies' websites because it makes the most money for them, as it keeps your children using diapers for a longer time. The idea is that you don't do anything to encourage nighttime dryness. You simply wait until they wake up dry.

   According to a study in *Pediatrics in Review*, 85 percent of the general population gains nighttime dryness by age 6. By doing nothing

SOMETHING TO KNOW BEFORE YOU START NIGHT TRAINING:

Know whether your child is peeing before falling asleep or between sleep cycles during the night. About 10 minutes after your child falls asleep, go check to see if their diaper feels full of urine. If the diaper is squishy from urine or warm to the touch, you can be pretty sure that your child probably peed right before falling asleep. If this is happening, focus your efforts on establishing a good nighttime routine of pottying and actually voiding just *before* bed. Sometimes incorporating a bath into a nighttime routine can relax a child and improve pottying efforts after the bath.

and providing a comfortable backup, there's no motivation for your child to learn bladder control. It can be harder to train children who are so thoroughly used to peeing in a diaper just before they go to bed. You can try this if you are trying to get through a season and need to ensure sleep.

I don't recommend this as a potty training method; I recommend it as a parental sleep method. For example, if a mother is pregnant or has a new baby, or a dad hurt his back and can't help, this is a way to maintain the level of wetness your child has at night. It is not an effective method to actually train your child to have nighttime dryness.

4. SWITCH TO UNDERWEAR AND JUST CHANGE SHEETS AND UNDIES UPON WETNESS, OR WHEN THEY CRY OR CALL OUT (NOT RECOMMENDED): I know many clients who tried this method before coming to me and were surprised when it didn't work for them. Basically, you've trained your child into diapers and this method gives them the full responsibility of training out of diapers, without any instruction. I don't recommend this method.

HOW TO NAP-TIME TRAIN

From my perspective, there is far more nervousness about nap training than there needs to be. Often nap training at the same time as day awake training is incredibly successful. I highly recommend trying to awake and nap train at the same time. I suggest this so that your child won't save their pee or poo for the diaper you give them at nap time. Additionally, telling your child that you're done with diapers is a lot easier to keep saying if they don't actually see one during the daytime.

If you do want to use a diaper or Pull-Up-like option, I recommend going with cloth so that your child can better feel the wetness. If your child is at preschool, they may require some sort of wetness barrier, so using rubber pants or something like Super Undies might be your best bet for preschool nap training that is still in the learning stage. If your child is in, or will soon be going to, preschool or day care, try to match your nap and pottying schedule to theirs the best that you can ahead of starting to day train, if possible.

SAMPLE NAP SCHEDULE:

Lunch: 11:30 a.m. to 12:00 p.m.

Take a trip to the potty with the goal of peeing first and then pooping: 12:00 p.m. to 12:30 p.m.

If they don't poop at the above potty trip, you can try adding in one more activity and one more potty trip, then straight to nap.

Nap: 12:30 p.m. to 2:00 p.m.

Upon waking, take your child to the bathroom sometime between immediately waking and within 20 minutes.

FAQ

Do I have to night train my child?

No, you don't. You can choose to skip this stage completely and just wait until their overnight diaper comes up dry. The catch is that waiting for dryness to happen doesn't actually teach your child how to use the bathroom during the night.

Walking to the bathroom alone in the dark can be a pretty scary thing, especially to a child who potentially hasn't ever been allowed out of their bed at night. It might just be scary enough to want to stay in bed and pee in the diaper they're used to. By showing your child what's expected of them (even in the night), you can help calm their fears and give them an example of what to do that they can learn to follow.

How do I take my child potty during the night?

You have a few options:

- You can physically pick your child up, hold them, and walk them to the toilet.
- You can have them walk to the toilet, while guiding them.
- You can have them walk to the toilet, independently.
- You can put a mini potty in their room, next to their bed, and have them go whenever they need to.

Do I have to wake my child up in order to take them during the night?

Not necessarily. You can try to "dream pee" them and place them on a mini potty or toilet without waking them fully.

How common is bedwetting?

According to the American Academy of Pediatrics, about 15 percent of six-year-old children wet their bed.

How do I know if my child has a bedwetting problem?

According to the National Institutes of Health National Institute of Diabetes and Digestive and Kidney Diseases, "By age 4, when most children stay dry during the day, daytime wetting can be very upsetting and embarrassing. By ages 5 or 6, children might have a bedwetting problem if the bed is wet once or twice a week over a few months."

If my child is still not staying dry during the night or after a nap even after trying the above methods, what can I do?

There are a few things you can try. You can try more frequent waking. You can try constipation remedies. You can attempt to reduce liquids

Ask a Parent

How did you handle nighttime, napping, and potty training?

"My son decided to not wear diapers and hasn't had an accident since (2 years and 8 months old). My other son was about the same age. I noticed his diapers always being dry and so I decided he was ready. Also, never an accident." —JAMES

"I would say she was nighttime trained way before she was actually [daytime] potty trained. She has never really been an overnight pee-er. So, I'll say from the first night we stopped diapers." —JUNE

"I've been told to cut liquids two hours before bed for nighttime/training, and for nap I just usually have my little guy go potty before and he stays dry the two hours he's asleep." —RUTH

A Note from Jennifer Singer, MD

Bedwetting is generally considered normal until about age 7. There is a tendency for bedwetting to run in families. Rarely is bedwetting related to an organic bladder dysfunction, though it can be. Isolated bedwetting beyond an acceptable age is generally considered a sleep disorder or disruption sometimes related to sleep apnea, tonsillar or adenoidal hypertrophy, or sleep patterns that have been disrupted for other reasons. Nighttime bladder control is a developmental process partly related to brain maturity. It occurs when the brain and bladder are ready, happening in response to signals transmitted through the spinal cord that the bladder is filling or full. In my practice, I use a variety of methods based on each child's individual circumstances. I do not recommend parental waking to time bathroom visits. I generally recommend limiting fluids two hours before bedtime when possible and voiding just prior to settling in. I often recommend a specialized bedwetting alarm system and, if appropriate, medication options can also be considered. There are also other approaches to bedwetting that are beyond the scope of this book. I encourage you to consider which approach may best fit the needs of your child and your family. If all options have failed, consulting with your physician is a good idea.

before bed. You can try cutting dairy out of their diet and switching to something like camel's milk, soy milk, or almond milk.

If none of those things work, there are exercises you can try for bladder control. There are conversations you can have with your child if accidents seem to happen when they are falling asleep, instead of during the course of the night. You can try co-sleeping so that you notice movements. Use your best judgment, as the safety of co-sleeping is debatable. You can choose to wait for a few weeks and try again. You can also seek medical help (see Chapter 13: Seeking Help, page 142).

EIGHT

Out and About

UNFAMILIAR ENVIRONMENTS

It's very likely that your child will encounter some unfamiliar environments just after potty training. They may not be used to going into a public restroom or may not know which is the kid-friendly bathroom at a friend's house. There are rules and expectations they have never experienced before. Though the mantra for potty training is to normalize for unfamiliar experiences, it's also to sympathize.

Yes, this is new. Yes, this is different. Yes, it may take some time to get used to it. But you know they can do it! You'll be there to comfort, reassure, and guide them each step of the way. In order to avoid extra unfamiliar environments, consider taking tours of common places, like your child's day care or preschool, their grandparents' house, favorite restaurants, and indoor playgrounds that you frequent, in advance to learn where their toilets are and what sort of child-friendly accommodations they have.

What Should I Bring with Me When I Leave the House?

Here is a list of items to consider bringing with you when you venture into unfamiliar environments:

- A complete change of clothes for your child, from head to toe. You'd be surprised what can get messy during some toddler accidents. This can include a hat, a shirt, a pair of pants, underwear, socks, shoes, and a jacket. I also recommend an extra set of the following: shirt, pants, underwear, and socks.
- A change of clothes for you in the trunk of your car (ideally including must-haves like shoes, a bra, etc.)
- Baby wipes
- Hand sanitizer or natural alternative (it's amazing how often accidents happen when you're nowhere near running water)
- Wet bag or plastic bag for soiled clothes
- Toilet paper/flushable wipes (just in case!)
- Rewards (if you're motivating extrinsically)
- Travel potty (optional to some, but essential to me!)
- Optional:
  - Sippy cup
  - Seat reducer
  - Seat covers for public toilets
  - Fiber-rich snack
  - Lysol spray or disinfectant

WHAT YOUR CHILD IS FEELING RIGHT NOW

If I were to guess, your child is actually far more confident about going out in undies than you are about them doing so. That may not be true, but typically it's *us*, as the parents, who are worried about their success, not them. If they've been stuck inside for a few days in a row, then they're probably more than ready to stretch their legs and get some fresh air!

Upon leaving the house they may be filled with nothing but confidence, but that may be short-lived. Once they learn that being potty trained means no longer using a changing table or being changed in the car, they may start to show their true colors. For many children, it starts upon the first mention of using a potty away from home. I recommend not mentioning toilets before you actually encounter one. Don't say anything until you see a toilet and know it's available for them to use. Then, mention that it's time to potty or you may have an accident along the way. Don't worry, it has happened on my watch!

Realize that your child may be scared to pee or poo away from the house. It's very common for this to happen. Keep in mind that many adults don't feel comfortable peeing and especially pooping away from the home. Your job is just to make needing to use a restroom away from the house feel normal, and part of the growing-up process.

FAQ

When should I start leaving the house?

As a general rule, when you feel ready to, or when your child can get at least half, ideally three fourths of their pees and poos in the toilet. I'm guessing the success will actually come before your confidence level, since we often adjust our confidence levels based on our views of success and failure.

I'm afraid my undies-clad child is going to pee in the car seat. What do I do?

You prepare as though you really, really don't want to wash that car seat . . . because you don't. Taking apart most car seats is a beast of a job! Take your child to the potty immediately before leaving the house. Offer the use of a travel potty upon arriving to the car. Put them in the car seat, and make sure it's lined. Lined can mean anything from a do-it-yourself water-absorbing burp cloth that's cut around the straps to a purchased waterproof, absorbent car seat insert (see Chapter 3: Are You Ready? on page 30 for a list of suggestions). Tell your child to tell you loudly if they need to go potty. Be willing to pull over and use a travel potty, if necessary.

My child is afraid of automatic public toilets. How can I get them to use them?

It's okay for your child to be scared. Prepare your child for the sounds and smells. You can often turn fear into laughter if you play along with them being scared and then break into laughter (not at your child, but at the situation). Are the automatic toilets loud and scary? Show a surprised face with your child, and then a crazy, silly face. Laughter is an amazing remedy for fear, as long as you're not laughing at your child's fear. Also, grab some Post-its and put them over the toilet sensor so that it doesn't flush while your child is still on the toilet and scare them out of peeing or pooping.

I don't want to haul around a toilet seat reducer. How do I get my child to feel comfortable on a public, friend's, or family member's toilet?

First things first: Has your child ever tried pottying without a toilet seat reducer at home? That might be worth a shot first. I suggest putting smaller-bottomed and younger kids backward on a toilet seat, facing the tank. That way they have more actual toilet seat supporting their bottom, rather than the falling-in feeling where they cling to the sides for dear life. If they do still want to face forward, have them spread their legs out as wide as possible to provide more support for themselves.

Any advice on flying? Would you do Pull-Ups for the flight, just in case?

What I personally would do is reserve seats at the back of the plane (next to the bathroom), bring a travel potty for good measure, and put a diaper on around the regular undies (but only while on the plane). I would take it off while in any airports and just camp out within quick walking distance of the public restroom.

Take your child to the bathroom at every opportunity possible before getting on and just after getting off a plane. Tell them ahead of time that the diaper is *only* for the flight and make it only for the flight—you might even make a special trip to the bathroom after landing just to take that diaper off and throw it in the trash (even if it's dry, just to make the point). You don't want your child forming any sort of attachment to it whatsoever.

Ask a Parent

How do you handle potty training outside of your home?

"The only way I've gotten my son to pee or poop while we are out of the house was not give him the option of a Pull-Ups or diaper. He wore shorts one day and the second day it was cold so he wore underpants and a pair of slacks. We've only tried going out without a diaper twice now but both days were successful and one of the days he did poop in a public restroom." —JANE

"I've had some success going out when we bring a portable seat and just bringing a towel, plastic bag, and a change of clothes, but also my kid responds just fine to a Pull-Ups on over her usual undies for longer trips. She can still feel the wetness of her undies if she goes. But I also let her pick her Pull-Ups (princess ones) just like she picked her (Peppa Pig) undies, and on days where she wears both, she says she doesn't want to get Peppa or Cinderella wet and she holds it! Worth a shot!" —ANDREW

NINE

Family and Other Caregivers

YOUR POTTY TRAINING TEAM

Teaching your child to successfully potty both at home and out and about is a common problem for many parents. I have had so very many consultations about the various details of this question. Many of the questions really boil down to, "How do I get my child who uses the potty at home to potty at preschool or out and about?" Or the opposite, "How do I get my child who uses the potty at preschool or out and about to potty at home?"

If you're dealing with this issue, you are not alone. With proper planning and practice, it can nearly always be handled. The basic idea you want them to learn is that toilets are for going potty in, when they feel they need to or when you or a caregiver tell them to, wherever they are. So how do you do this? The main thing is communication.

What to Communicate to Caregivers

You want to get everyone on board with your potty training plan and give them the information and resources they need to make this happen. At the same time, you need to be open to them telling you what they're doing; if you have been entrusting your child to someone else's care a bulk of the day, they are your co-parent, too. Here is what you should provide and go over with them:

- Give them a copy of this plan, tailored to your family.
- Tell them where you're at on the plan and what your next step is.
- Give them an ideal time line for the overall plan.
- Give them the tools to make it happen.
- Talk about what your plan is for naps and nights.
- Discuss the use of overnight diapers and diapers that pull on, whether they be disposable or cloth.
- Be aware of what their "they can't come back" policy is. Often it's a "two strikes they're out" rule.

A great potty training practice to have is to try to have your family's home schedule mimic your child's preschool or day care schedule for a little while. If your child is spending two to five days during their main awake hours out of your care, then you need to take into consideration that for your child it may not actually feel normal to play by your rules. You are the parent and you do get the final say, but to some degree you have decided to share your parenting responsibilities with another care provider. For your child's best success, you need to try to establish one "normal."

That said, typically you do not need to turn leisurely life on a Saturday into another day of preschool. Far from it—go on a walk, visit a relative, or head to the beach or the mountains. But when you are first trying to get potty training down, it is important to maintain a routine and some structure to your day, so as not to confuse your child.

Your preschool will reinforce what you are teaching about potty train-ing, and you will reinforce what your preschool is teaching about potty training. It will be a beautifully clear plan for your child.

Mirror Your Preschool's Pottying Schedule and Routine

Within reason, try to mirror your child's preschool routine at home within 15-minute intervals. On the next page, you'll find a sample schedule.

TRY TO MIMIC THINGS FROM PRESCHOOL

Schedule: Match up times of the day as best you can, or at least the flow of the preschool's routine, which, for potty training purposes, tends to revolve mostly around snacks and lunch.

What they sit on: If the potty at school is actually the toilet, then mirror by having them use a toilet at home as well.

Their position: If they face backward at preschool toward the tank, have them do that at home as well.

Make the transition from home to preschool as simple as possible by eliminating all of the surprise factors.

FAQ

It doesn't matter what I take away, my child will never initiate to go to the bathroom on their own. It has become a problem at preschool; when the teachers ask them to go, they always say no. What can I do?

Be very clear. Ask all other care providers to be on the same page with you. That means anything from a spouse or co-parent, to preschool, to church, to a mother-in-law. Tell them all that you need your child to be *told* it is time to go to the bathroom. Tell them you don't want your child being *asked*, but would like your child being told that it is potty time, and then have them taken.

SCHEDULING AT HOME AND AWAY

PRESCHOOL/CHILD CARE	HOME
Not applicable	____A.M. Take child to the bathroom within first 5 to 10 minutes of waking (or at least within 20 minutes of waking)
Not applicable	___A.M. Take after breakfast when the feeling of being "full" is to your advantage
8:15 A.M. Takes potty upon arrival to preschool	8 A.M.–8:30 A.M. Take at whatever time they would normally get to school
10:15 A.M. 15-minute snack time followed by a potty trip	10:00 A.M.–10:30 A.M. 15-minute snack time followed by a potty trip
10:30 A.M. Potty trip (uses a regular-sized toilet)	10:15 A.M.–10:45 A.M. Potty trip (if possible, use whatever sort of toilet they use at preschool)
11:00 A.M. 30-minute lunch	10:45 A.M.–11:15 A.M. 30-minute lunch
11:30 A.M. All students taken to the potty	11:15 A.M.–11:45 A.M. Take to the potty
2:00 P.M. 15-minute snack time followed by a potty trip	1:45 P.M.–2:15 P.M. 15-minute snack time followed by a potty trip
3:00 P.M. Pickup time	2:45 P.M.–3:15 P.M. Either take to the potty at this time or offer at this time, and then take upon returning home or arriving at their next activity

My mother-in-law keeps guilt-tripping me and saying that it's well past time to potty train my child because her kids could all use the toilet by age 1. Is she right?

It sounds like you're feeling judged. I'm sorry that's happening. My number one thought is to learn what you can from her input, and forget the rest. She thinks your child is able, and she thinks that if you try to, you are able to teach your child to use the potty. Those are both encouraging! She very well may never have potty trained but actually practiced elimination communication, which is a whole different ball game.

Also take into consideration the context she trained in. She very well may have lived with lots of help nearby, in a culture of early potty learning, or in a society where disposable diapers weren't normal. Don't sweat it. From her perspective, I'm guessing she just wants what she thinks is best for her grandchildren. You want the best for your child, too; it just may play out differently for your family.

My relative demands that I put my child in a diaper/Pull-Ups at their house because they don't believe my child could be potty trained yet. How should I respond?

As a courtesy to others, I tend to lean toward "their house, their rules." You can always choose not to go to their house. But if there are reasons that you strongly want to be there while potty training, or just after potty success, and others aren't comfortable with your child out of a diaper, figure out the situation that they would be comfortable with.

Is it really that they are nervous about their new couch? Maybe the solution would be to have your child sit on the floor. Are they worried about carpeting? Bring over a piddle pad, or a small tarp and put a blanket on top. Once they see the effort you are going to, and that accidents aren't happening, they'll probably back down. After all, "seeing is believing." If they haven't seen your child's potty training success, they probably don't believe it's real yet.

My child is stuck in the two-year-olds' class because they aren't potty trained. I don't want them held back educationally just because they still use a diaper. What can I do?

First of all, no shame in where you're at. Just start from there. Try your best not to reflect your own emotions (fear of failure? embarrassment?) on your child.

Secondly, voice your concerns to your preschool director and let staff know that you're ready to potty train. Do the initial work at home, and then let them know you would like, and expect, them to maintain the work you've started by moving your child into a class where pottying is expected. Be clear that you don't want your child to be asked if they need to go; instead, you want them to be told when it's time to go.

As far as education goes, most kids can catch up in a flash. They are sponges, just waiting to soak up new experiences and facts about the world around them. Keep egging on their curiosity about the world in general by encouraging their questions and observations, such as "I wonder . . ." and "I notice . . . ," and they'll be fine as far as learning goes.

My child's preschool wants to potty train my child, but I don't think I'm ready to follow up at home. Should I tell them not to? Or should I let them potty train at preschool, but put my child in diapers at home?

I believe that in the long term, any potty learning is better than none. But take into consideration that if you potty train at preschool and not at home, it's likely that if there are accidents in the future, then the bulk of the accidents will probably be with the less familiar pottying environment. Since that could be your home, you may choose not to potty train until you can do it all at the same time. However, I recommend making the best of someone else's investing in your child's progress. Feel free to ask them their rationale. Note that they should respect your decision, whichever decision you choose, and I support you whatever you decide as well.

My child has split custody and spends half their time at my ex's. My ex doesn't want to potty train, but I do. How should I handle this?

The answer to this is similar to the preceding preschool-versus-home question. Some potty training is better than none, but it's likely that the bulk of potential future accidents will be in the home your child is less familiar pottying in. Again, you might want to try asking your ex their rationale.

Ask a Parent

This Ask a Parent question comes from Jane: "My son has been completely potty trained for about a month but he has never been with anyone else but me and his dad. When I went to the day care today, they said maybe put him in Pull-Ups in case he had accidents, but I don't want to do that. He has not had an accident in over three weeks. HELP!"

"I wouldn't do it. That could make him go backwards. Just send extra clothes with him (socks, underwear, pants, and shirt). My two are in preschool, my oldest is potty trained and I send extra clothes with him." —LISA

"I'd tell them no. If they can't help, then tell them you will be seeking an alternative to them." —THERESA

"Treat him like he is potty trained. If he has an accident, then they change him and move on. Day cares should expect that." —SARAH

Here's another Ask a Parent question, from Deborah: "My son has been having accidents every time I pick him up. Sometimes his teachers don't even realize it because it's at story time, which is the last thing they do. He's so timid and shy at school that unless they do potty time, he won't tell them. I'm not sure what to do. I think if he went right before story time that he would be okay, but I know it's hard on his teachers to ask them to do something special. He really likes school and they haven't acted like they care, but I would love to help fix the problem. Any ideas?! Thank you!"

"Tell his teachers to ask him to go before story time to avoid accidents." —GERALDINE

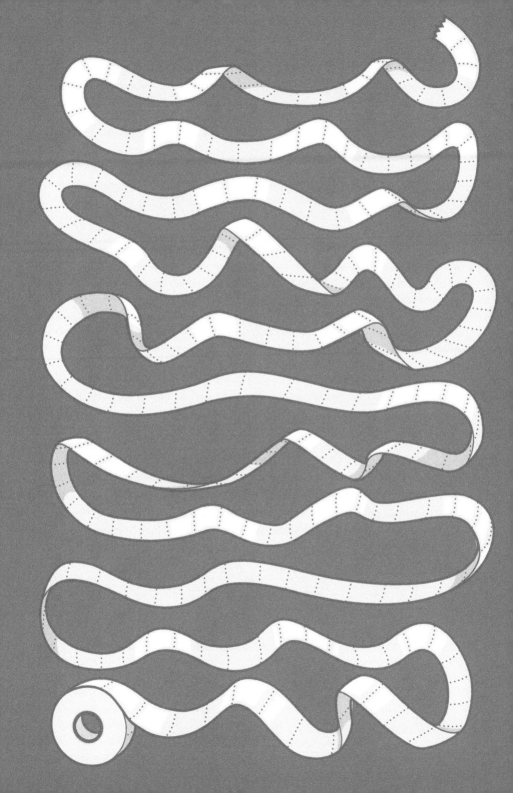

Part Three

FURTHER HELP AND ADVICE

Common Resistance Behavior

Special Circumstances

Accidents and Backsliding

Seeking Help

TEN

Common Resistance Behavior

WHEN YOUR CHILD SAYS NO

You've asked your child if they need to go potty and they said, "No." Big surprise, right? If your child can indicate a "no" response, at some point they are most probably going to resist using the potty. It is a very, very common problem. One way of avoiding this battle is to teach pottying before your child learns to say no as a means of resistance, which happens at about 13 months.

But if you haven't done that, what can you do?

The phase of habitual no's is mostly about human nature. Once a child can resist, they will. They're learning what's within their sphere of influence to control. It's a matter of power. According to Barbara K. Polland, PhD, author of *No Directions on the Package*, you child starts saying no because "they're discovering that they can make their own decisions." They want to have the power. What are you to do?

You weigh the benefits for them and make a loving decision on their behalf. You never asked if they wanted to sit in a car seat, but you strap them in every day because you can see both the short-term and long-term benefits.

How Are *You* Resisting?

Are you being the biggest resistance problem to your potty training journey? Are you the one

- Procrastinating?
- Expecting immediate gratification?
- Fearful?
- Projecting your emotions on your child?
- Criticizing or doubting yourself?
- Experiencing a paralysis of analysis (being overwhelmed by figuring out what to do with all the information)?

Take a minute to do a quick self-check at how you may be adding to the resistance equation.

Why and How Your Child Is Resisting

According to Edward Teyber and Faith Teyber's *Interpersonal Process in Therapy: An Integrative Model*, "The common source of resistance and defenses is shame." Let's explore why and how your child is resisting potty training so we can help them overcome.

Mentally: It could be a range of thoughts. Anything from shame manifested as self-doubt to perfectionism manifested as people-pleasing. They might want to be seen as independent and invulnerable, or want to withdraw socially.

Physically: Sometimes kids will go to extremes to push back physically. Common resistance behaviors include running away, throwing themselves on the ground, throwing items, pushing, hitting, or crying. Please don't treat these behaviors as acceptable. You will have to teach your child not to do these things.

Emotionally: Generally speaking, there are various types of pleas, like crying, manipulating, and bargaining. Don't teach your child this behavior.

Stating the facts: Don't let your child tell you what their perception of reality is. You will often hear phrases like "I just went," "I would rather use a diaper," or "I don't have to go now." This is just another way for them to say no and resist.

How to Overcome Resistance

It all comes back to normalizing the potty. Human brains are equipped to overcome resistance. It may not feel like it when your toddler fights with every ounce of their body weight, but it *is* possible. For example, when you tell your child they get to learn to use the potty, they probably react in one of two ways. The first reaction is that they think it's a good idea and your child's brain releases feel-good neurotransmitters. The other reaction is that they think it's a bad idea and they create barriers in their mind that help validate why it is bad and why they should avoid it.

But it doesn't have to end there. We can teach our children to get out of their own way by helping them reframe how they think about the situation. Maybe they don't like the idea because they don't want to be a big girl or big boy. Sometimes the fix is as easy as focusing on something else. If your child is viewing potty training as an imposition in their life, reframe it for them as a positive addition that allows for things like freedom, independence, and new undies. You can start reframing your child's resistance into something that will actually add to the pottying journey, instead of taking away from it.

Picture a toddler who has no concept of using the potty. You casually walk down the aisle of a hardware store and point out that the potties are "for pee pee and poo poo" and continue walking. Then maybe another time you mention that as soon as you get to Grandma's house and before you leave, you use the toilet. After time, if we start exemplifying to our children that using the potty is normal, they will actually start noticing

WHAT YOUR CHILD IS FEELING RIGHT NOW

Your child is feeling three primary things right now. They are annoyed, they are frustrated, and they want more control. If you're reading this chapter, it's pretty likely that you are feeling these things, too.

Annoyed: *Your child may be a little annoyed at your pestering them about using the potty or being wet or dry. They may just be sick of the whole conversation. If this is the case, try to stop talking. Try to listen. Try to teach by showing. Talk less, listen more.*

Frustrated: *Maybe your child is legitimately trying and is frustrated for not saying something in time to avoid an accident. Or maybe they're frustrated that they have to keep stopping playing in order to get their clothes changed. If this is the case, try your best to empathize with them. Do not validate the accidents; validate the feelings. You don't need to say, "It's okay that you wet yourself." Instead say, "You look frustrated that you wet yourself. It's okay to feel frustrated. How can I help?"*

Wanting more control: *I would be surprised if this is not the main issue happening. Often children resist because there is some part of the process that they want control over in which you keep bossing them around. For this, give them more responsibility. Let them help (at least in part, ideally fully) with anything and everything they want to, even if it means a bit more time or mess. In the long term it will be truly efficient to your overall journey.*

more often than before that people are using the potty, which will help normalize it for them. Human beings can let in only so many new ideas. But once we let an idea in, we make connections to the world through that idea. Bank on that natural process by normalizing the potty, instead of forcing a child to use it.

FAQ

How do I get my child to sit on the potty?

To be blunt, this is the wrong perspective. The goal is not to get your child to sit on the toilet. The end goal is to get them to put their pee and poo in the potty, and that doesn't happen by sitting on the potty. Getting your child to sit for long periods might actually have the opposite effect when it comes time to actually getting that pee or poo in the potty!

However, if it's a matter of sitting on the potty when they need to go, often moving from the mini potty up to the regular toilet on a seat reducer can help. Or if they're sitting forward on the toilet and they're popping off, facing them backward can help delay them.

Why does my child sit on the potty, pee one drop, and then have an accident five minutes later?

It's very likely somehow your child has been trained to sit on the toilet in order to please you, or to gratify themselves, instead of to actually use it. They quite probably are in the habit of sitting on the toilet because you cheer them on, or because you give them something. You need to break this association of "pottying = getting something."

I'd encourage taking away all the prizes and having some naked or half-naked time at home. Then if they have an accident, have them help you clean up (either up close and personal with the accident or from a distance—your decision).

How do you motivate your child when none of the other tools and tricks work?

Stop trying to motivate them. Seriously, stop trying to convince them. Just show them how to do it. Take them with you. Normalize the process. If you really feel like you've tried every possible option, then you yourself just might need to take a break for a few days and start up again after you've had more than three consecutive conversations that didn't involve talking about potty training woes. It might be that you need a break more than your child does.

My child just doesn't want to use the toilet. They earnestly *want* to pee or poo in their diaper. Is it mean to potty train them when they so obviously prefer their diaper?

If we step back and look at the overall goal, it would be counterproductive to allow that. Remember the cognitive reframing we talked about earlier in the book? This is where it plays out. Work on trying to reframe the benefits of teaching your child to put their pee or poo in the toilet.

Everyone keeps telling me to take a break and that it will help with the resistance problems, but I'm afraid it will do more harm than good. Advice?

If the person who needs the break is you, then I wholeheartedly encourage you to take a break. Whether it's life, or feeling like you can't keep going, or just needing some time for encouragement, it's okay to take a break. But note that it's very likely that starting back up again will actually lead to *more* resistance, and more of a battle of the wills.

If the person who needs the break is your child, then I encourage you to stay with it. Maybe that sounds mean, but you need to guide your child to what is most helpful for them. They can't see the greater good; you can. If they're resistant because of something like having had diarrhea or constipation and they don't want to use the toilet because of a fear that it will hurt, address the fear. Be there with them in their fear, but don't stop the overall game plan because of it.

Ask a Parent

What do you do when your child resists potty training?

"The first three to five days look very hopeless, but it does get better. Keep going, don't give up! For the first few days, rush him on the potty as soon as you see him pee or poo and say, 'Pee or poo goes in the potty.' You'll also learn his frequency. After the first few days, he'll know where he's supposed to go and you'll know his frequency so you can take him to the potty every X minutes. Do something he finds interesting while he's on the toilet. For my son, it's reading. He picked out a bunch of books. I have a bin of them in the bathroom. Most importantly, don't give up, keep going. You got this.

Distract him with his subject/object of interest, so that he doesn't mind being taken to the potty. Sit him on the toilet. He'll most likely finish peeing without even knowing, since he's distracted. If not, remind him gently to pee.

If this fails, let him pee on the floor. Remind him that it's the wrong place for the pee. Have him help you clean up. As he is helping you, explain how much work it is to clean up. But if he went in the potty, there would be no clean up, and he gets to flush! Tell him how feeling wet is none too awesome. Make your best 'yucky' face. Tell him that grown-ups go in the potty. It'll look hopeless today and tomorrow. But he'll learn. He IS learning, this is how he learns." —DEANNA

"I took a break for a few months. The breaks really help I think! Helps everyone regroup." —SOPHIA

"Our pediatrician told us to take a break and let him go back into diapers as [our son's resistance] was most likely caused by stress. We are going to try again later." —REBECCA

ELEVEN

Special Circumstances

I push aside the things that I generally teach and pull out the whole bag of tricks for special-needs and special-circumstances children. I want you to be open to something outside the norm of how society typically teaches potty training and be willing to pursue methods that work in other cultures, even if it's uncomfortable for you.

I am not a doctor, but cultural differences about toilet training are influencing many doctors, per an article in the *Canadian Medical Association Journal* titled "Toilet Training Children: When to Start and How to Train." The article actually says toilet training is a "complex process that can be affected by anatomic, physiologic and behavioral conditions. Accepted norms of toilet training relate more to cultural differences than scientific evidence. Despite this, parents continue to approach their family physicians and pediatricians for advice about toilet training."

That said, I'm honored to be of service to you as well.

DEVELOPMENTAL ISSUES

When it comes to special needs, I am very willing to cross cultural borders of norms, and I don't assume your child fits into any previous child's journey. We often need to try something new or slightly different. Use what they *are* able to do, even if that's simply grunting or moving one arm. You can teach communication. If you need some inspiration, learn about deaf-blind woman Helen Keller and her teacher, Annie Sullivan. You will be humbled and encouraged at how we can learn to use our other senses, and how love and commitment can make all the difference.

For the sake of this chapter, we'll say there are three areas of development that can affect your potty training:

1. SPEECH (receptive and expressive)

2. MOTOR SKILLS (gross motor and fine motor)

3. SOCIAL AND EMOTIONAL AWARENESS

Speech

If you are willing to adjust your idea of potty training to include partial words or hand signals, then let's make this work. You will have more work than the average speech-developed child's parent because you will need to help your child identify when they feel the urge to go, and teach them how to convey that to you through partially developed or lacking word usage.

My husband and I know firsthand that this plan works with an expressively speech-delayed child because we used it with our speech-delayed daughter. At the time, she couldn't even do the proper hand signals. Somehow, we managed, and even convinced caregivers to recognize her ability to communicate her need to potty.

Talk with your speech pathologist for ideas of which words to use. Don't be disheartened if your speech therapist tells you your child isn't ready and you should "wait" until they are (refer to Chapter 2: Is Your

Child Ready?, page 13). You are the parent, and you get to decide if your family is ready to start potty training, speech delay or not.

If your child is speech delayed, try to incorporate some of the following into your potty training routine:

- Hand signals (gestures)
- Sounds that aren't words (partial words, vowel sounds, grunts, etc.)
- Picture cards or photos
- A speech-generating device
- Sense of smell (to recognize pee or poo)
- Responding to sounds they hear
- Use the word *potty* instead of *toilet* (p's typically develop before t's)

Motor Skills

Gross Motor: It is likely that you may have a fully potty-able child who is never able to get onto the toilet themselves. You may always need to take them. For those with children who have severe cerebral palsy, for example, it is likely that you may need to just focus on poop training for the first few months.

Fine Motor: It *is* possible to have a fully potty-able child who can't unbutton their pants or wash their hands on their own. As long as they're getting their pee and poo in the right place, that's the win! Focus on what they can accomplish. Maybe at first, they aren't able to turn the light on, but after time they can. Or perhaps flushing the toilet takes two hands and a full-body effort. Commend the hard work!

Social and Emotional Skills

Social Skills: A child who lacks the ability to notice the social climate around them isn't going to be influenced much by normalizing the potty. It doesn't impact them the way it does other children, and that's okay. In their case, you should aim to be practical, demonstrative, and visual. The fact that other children use the potty and your child uses a diaper doesn't matter to your child. But going on a tour of a new bathroom and going through all the pieces of the pottying puzzle tend to make much more sense. Show them what to do, step by step. Have printouts up in the bathroom areas. Have them take cues from the surroundings and schedule of the day, rather than using social cues. Emphasize wet and dry, and have them feel and touch to learn the difference between the two. Using light-colored underwear can make it more obvious when their underwear is wet, so that's worth a try as well. Pottying watches can also be helpful with socially delayed children.

BELIEVE IN YOUR CHILD

Having a child with special circumstances can be _____, _____, and _____. [Please fill in the blanks.]

I know that *you* know better than I do how that can feel with your child in particular. Potty training on its own can feel like a huge milestone and can be even more daunting to the parent with special circumstances to deal with as well. I implore you to lean on the side of believing that your child can do it. That doesn't mean you should make your nonverbal child talk or your autistic child initiate on the first day. But it does mean that if people tell you something's impossible, you should seek the tiny parts of the process that might be possible for your child if modified. You and your child's team of caregivers know your child best. Believe in your child. Trust what your gut is telling you they can achieve. As my husband often says, "I choose to believe the best in people." I encourage you to do the same.

Emotional Skills: For children who are emotionally delayed, you are probably firmly aware that even if they *can* talk, often they choose not to because of the unwanted attention given to them. Or it may be the complete opposite: They just talk and talk, but would never mention they need to go to the bathroom. For the sake of potty training, I'd recommend reviewing (and potentially talking to a behavioral therapist) which skills your child has as a solid foundation, and bank on those. If your child is good at using picture cards, use those. If they can use a light to signal a need, use that. Don't expect your child to ask a class attendant to take them to the bathroom; tell the attendant that your child needs to be taken. If needed, it's perfectly okay to focus on mastering pottying at home for a few weeks before trying it at preschool or day care. Feel free to tell staff that you would like to be present during the first day back at class to help with any transitions your child may need assistance with. Though time-consuming, it's much less of an imposition than if your child has continuous accidents and you get called in day after day to pick your child up from school.

LIFE CHANGES

It's easy to assume any sort of change will disrupt potty training. People blame anything, like getting molars, a new sibling, moving, a food allergy, or alterations in sleep patterns. Parents, let's be realistic. Life is going to happen. You can't halt your parenting efforts upon every change that comes your way. Children will be affected in different ways. For one child, moving might be a hard change because they spend most of the time on the first floor of an apartment and the toilet is now on the second floor. For another, a move may allow them to quickly run inside from outdoor play, reducing accidents.

My encouragement is to keep trekking and see how things go, unless you have planned travel. In that case, try to start the process after returning from the trip.

If there is medical trauma, use your best discretion. In general, talk with someone you have confidence in to offer sound advice.

FAQ

Please accept my apologies if these answers seem trite. It is incredibly counterproductive to give one-size-fits-all advice to any family, let alone a family with a child with special needs. Special circumstances or developmental delays cover such a broad range of topics with both difficulties and joys. There is no way these answers can capture and express the desire I have to truly help your family. I only wish a few words on a page could adequately do that for you. But at least this will be a place that we can start together.

No one thinks my child is able to use the potty because of a developmental delay. But I don't think they've given my child a fair chance. What can I do?

First of all, I want you to know that I am completely on your side. In a world of naysayers doing what's easiest and most normal, specialists tend to stick to the party line in terms of what their patient is capable of. Unfortunately, sometimes that means that they fail to address and implement a plan to encourage pottying independence (or even lessen dependence upon diapers).

That said, you *can* fight for your child. You can fight most effectively by caring about those who are serving your child. Crazy thought, right? You need to tell them that you will support them and encourage them, and then do it! Along the way, follow through and speak (or write, potentially to a superior!) highly of them and their efforts whenever possible. Sing praises of how you feel like they are one of the few gems of a teacher, therapist, psychologist, or anyone else who is seeing what your child is truly capable of, and of how grateful you are of them. Also, take a quick review of Chapter 9: Family and Other Caregivers (page 108) and make sure you're all on the same page. More than anything, keep it positive. Make it worth their while for your child to succeed, or for your child to at least be given the chance.

My child is receiving ongoing services. I hate to stop my child's routine in order to potty train them. What is more effective: keeping them on their regular schedule or staying home for a bit to focus on potty training?

This is an excellent question. The true answer is that I don't know. If your child is particularly affected by a change in their schedule, like some children who have Down syndrome or autism can be, then I would encourage you to get caregivers on board throughout your week to help while maintaining your set schedule. Plan to have focused potty training time, potentially for two back-to-back weekends.

If it's really hard for your child to emotionally attach to people or to leave you, then it may be worthwhile to do the potty training at home and then ask to be involved in their class setting for a few days after training to help them transition to the new environment.

The answer is that both can be effective, or ineffective, depending on your child and the variables at play.

My child has a speech delay. How can I potty train them if they can't ever *say* that they need to go?

Fully potty trained children never, ever need to say, "I need to go potty, Mommy." One of our children had a speech delay and didn't associate "dada" with "Daddy" until she was 18 months old. But at 17 months she was fully out of diapers during the day and had weeks' worth of dry times before then. We mostly waited until 17 months for the sake of caregivers. Most of them thought we were nuts, except one: Melissa.

Melissa listened when I said that I believed children can learn to use the potty using their other senses. For us that meant finishing up elimination communication (which uses a sound association with the need to potty) and hand signals. At the time, our daughter was incapable of doing the standard signed and shaken *T* for "toilet" often used in American Sign Language, so she just shook her hand. When she first started this at about 11 months, people would wave back at her and she'd start crying. I'm convinced it's because she knew they didn't know what she meant.

With time, she made it so obvious that she needed to go, by grunting and waving her right hand with one finger pointed up, that caregivers started to ask if she was potty trained before we ever took off the diaper.

My child has so many people on their care team that I don't know whose "job" it is to potty train my child. Are they expecting me to do it all?

If your child has a care team, then your whole team needs to be involved. If your child is a year and a half or older, it would be very wise to start having conversations as to when and how different members of your child's care team think potty training "should" be done and how to go about it. You need to get on the same page as to *how* to be involved. You don't want one behavioral therapist taking your child alone to the toilet every 10 minutes while the aide at preschool takes the children in a big group every two hours. You want as much continuity as possible. You can definitely have a say as to both *when* and *how* they potty train as well. They do not need to be on a set schedule. If your child has a one-on-one aide, it is perfectly reasonable to ask the aide to look for signs that your child actually needs to go instead of just taking them every X minutes.

I'm a working parent. How can I use this plan if I can't take a few days off in a row to devote to potty training?

Be as dedicated as you can be, when you can be. If you have only a few hours at a time, make those few hours effective. Fill them with quality time with your child, but also pay as much attention as possible to any signs of their needing to potty.

The most surefire way to figure out quickly if your child is currently peeing or pooing is by seeing them. For those who have to potty train in increments, I highly recommend naked training. It will give your child an obvious "I am potty training" and "I am not potty training" differ-ence. Tell them when you are switching to not potty training, and explain that they are getting a diaper/Pull-Up, but that you still want them to put their pee and poo in the potty instead of their diaper. At any sign of needing to go, even when wearing a diaper, take them to the toilet with the same speed that you would if they weren't wearing a diaper.

Keep in mind, there's nothing magic about your starting day being on a weekend. Do it whenever you are able to. Props to you for doing what you can to provide for your child. I'm sure there's a lot of sacrifice involved already; no need to add guilt.

Ask a Parent

How do you potty train a child who has developmental issues?

"My son has autism and is practically nonverbal (only says a few clearly understandable words). We got him trained within a week, but still had an accident here or there for a few weeks. Then about a month later he totally regressed and would have multiple accidents a day. We didn't know what else to do so we just kept trying and about two weeks later he was back on track. Every now and then he still has accidents, but so would a child without autism. He's trained for both weeing and pooing on a toilet." —RALPH

"My four-and-half-year-old runs away from me and hits me about going to the potty. I looked up some information about autism by behavioral specialists. My three-and-half-year-old son is autistic and semi-nonverbal. He is just now starting to pee on the potty. It's hit or miss with him though. Some days he's up for it and some days he's not." —BRIAN

TWELVE

Accidents and Backsliding

ACCIDENTS HAPPEN

When you think you are done with messes, an accident can bring up a flurry of emotions. You are not alone. I can almost guarantee your child will have more than one accident. I can remember having a meeting to share my pottying wisdom as the CEO of The Potty School, when my already-potty-independent-no-accidents-for-two-months toddler walked in, pants quite obviously soaking wet, saying, "Potty!"

It was very humbling—a reminder that accidents happen to everyone.

When I went to go check out the scene I saw that she had taken the toy sink out of a kids' kitchen set and tried to use it as a toilet. It was on the floor, filled with urine. When I went to dump the potty in the regular bathroom I realized that the door was closed and she wasn't yet tall enough to open it.

Accidents will happen. But remember these two things:

1. YOU HAVE ACCIDENTS IN LIFE: When you fail, the last thing you want is someone to focus on what you did wrong. You want someone to teach you how to do it better next time and let you know that they still love and accept you. The same is true of our children. Don't just reassure them that the accident is okay. Recognize that it was an accident, and that they're learning. Encourage them to do better next time by being very specific in what you expect of them. Maybe you could say, "Next time you need to go potty, tell Mommy and I'll help you."

2. GO THE EXTRA MILE TO LEARN MORE ABOUT YOUR CHILD: If you pay attention, you can often easily learn why an accident is happening. Perhaps your child was distracted watching television, or maybe you forgot to stop and tell them it was potty time. Maybe they have on a Pull-Up and they didn't feel the wetness. With observation, there are often situations you can learn to avoid as well as behaviors that you actually can encourage. Perhaps they were on their way to the potty, or told you they needed to go potty, and then went immediately. Encourage that "telling ahead of time" behavior. Find what you can encourage and do so. Saying, "That's okay," is validating accidents. You don't want to normalize accidents; instead, you want them to learn from them.

Your Perspective about Accidents Matters

Those who don't have accidents haven't tried something new. Remembering what two of the greats have said about accidents over time might help give you some perspective on the how to view accidents as a whole.

"The ideal man bears the accidents of life with dignity and grace, making the best of circumstances." —ARISTOTLE

"I'm selfish, impatient, and a little insecure. I make mistakes, I am out of control, and at a times hard to handle. But if you can't handle me at my worst, then you sure . . . don't deserve me at my best." —MARILYN MONROE

When Accidents Become a Problem

Maybe your child was completely potty trained and they are starting to have accidents all of a sudden. Remember how I talked about how potty training ebbs and flows? Kids learn like a spiral curve. The overall learning is headed in an upward direction, but sometimes they're taking the long way to get there. That's okay. That's normal. Setbacks often do occur, but they're typically not a reason to give up. Keep at it.

"WHY DOESN'T MY CHILD JUST STOP AND GO TO THE BATHROOM?"

Answers to this question vary widely, and could include:

- Being too busy and focused on what they're doing
- Being lazy
- Physically not noticing (common with autistic kids)
- Being too embarrassed to ask to use the restroom
- Not caring about the implications
- Feeling uncomfortable to potty away from home
- Being blocked (constipation blockage)
- Diarrhea
- Medical conditions
- Psychological conditions (much more rare than medical causes)

Accidents are a fine dance between your child being diaper trained and being potty trained. Sometimes we take too much control; sometimes we give too much control. It's difficult to decide when a series of accidents has become a more serious trend that needs to be addressed without knowing more about your child and the patterns that are normal. Generally speaking, if you feel like you're on day one or day two of potty training all over again out of the blue and don't have an obvious cause (like a stomach bug), then it's worthwhile to seek help. An undiagnosed UTI is not fun for an adult, let alone a toddler. We'll talk more about when to seek outside help in the next chapter.

WHAT YOUR CHILD IS
FEELING RIGHT NOW

Accidents can be embarrassing for both child and parent. Whether it's while you're giving your friend tips on how you potty trained "so quickly" and your child has an accident that moment, or your child is running off to play with friends at a park and has to stop because they just wet their pants, accidents aren't fun.

Be patient with your child. If it is a true accident (unintentional) then just get them to the toilet or a travel potty to finish putting any more pee or poo in the potty. Then get them cleaned up (either let them help or not) and have them be on their way. Don't make a public spectacle about it. Don't bad-mouth your child's accident. Don't vent about potty training frustrations in front of them. They're probably already bummed to miss the next activity as it is. Point it out, but don't rub it in. That will do more harm than the accident itself.

You love your child *through* accidents, not despite them. The goal isn't just to potty train, but to have a loving, trusting relationship with your child—focus on that. Don't dwell on the accidents.

FAQ

I get so frustrated when my child has an accident! What should I do?

It is totally normal for you to get frustrated. We just have to make sure our reactions are kept in check. Accidents cause extra work for you. Accidents that are actually intentional can be super frustrating when children use it as a means of control. The best way to curb the control is by having them help with the cleanup in some way or another. Many parents get frustrated that their child isn't as fazed by the mess as they are. Level the playing field. Let them put some skin in the game and help with the mess, either by actually cleaning or by at least postponing whatever activity they are doing while you are cleaning up.

How many accidents are "normal" per day?

In the first few days of potty training, accidents are normal and to be expected. After the first few days, up to four accidents is still in the realm of normal. Most children shouldn't have more than one or two accidents a day past the first week if they are being taken at normal times throughout the day and given a routine of when to potty. That does *not* mean taking them every 30 minutes. It means taking them when they wake up, after meals, before leaving for somewhere, upon arrival, and so on. Please note: "Normal" doesn't mean this will apply to everyone. There are kids with autism who take to potty training better than most non-autistic kids. Most kids will still have an accident here or there for a few months if they're under age three. Just watch for your child's signs and try to keep a basic potty schedule.

For how long is it "normal" for a child to have accidents?

There is such huge variety in this answer and so many variables. Some kids don't have accidents past day one. For most, it's usually about one to two weeks and then every once in a while after then. It definitely depends on the child's age as well. A four-year-old usually won't have as many accidents as a two-year-old, generally speaking, because their bladder can hold a lot more and they physiologically don't need to void as often.

Do you consider bedwetting an accident? Or do you suggest dealing with it differently?

Bedwetting, as defined below, is a medical diagnosis. Bedwetting (nocturnal enuresis) should be dealt with separately from daytime potty training. According to *Pediatrics in Review,* a publication of the American Academy of Pediatrics, "Primary nocturnal enuresis (PNE) is defined as nocturnal [night time] wetting in a child who has never been dry on consecutive nights for longer than 6 months. It is estimated that between 5 and 7 million children and adolescents may suffer from this disorder. The incidence of PNE is based on age. Dryness is expected to be achieved by 5 years of age; if not, the child is diagnosed as having PNE."

I have people in my life who think it's not a big deal for my child to have accidents, but I feel like it's a backhanded way of telling me I'm not potty training correctly or my way is incorrect.

This makes total sense, from both perspectives. They're not in it like you are, but you don't have the perspective that they do. It's likely they're trying to extend grace to you, instead of condemning you. It's also possible that you're totally right and that it's a passive-aggressive way for them to express what they're thinking. If you're feeling threatened or offended, it would be best to talk to them about it (without your child present) instead of trying to guess what they meant, being offended by something they didn't mean, or avoiding it and having it put a wedge in your relationship.

How do I increase the amount of time between pottying?

For some children who thrive on complete structure, or physically have a hard time noticing that they need to void, a timed schedule can be helpful. But once your child has shown success approximately 75 percent of the time, it's reasonable to increase the duration between offers, increasing it an additional 15 minutes. You can do this from once a day to once every two days, depending on what you think your child is capable of. According to the article "Toilet Training Children with Autism Spectrum Disorders," you should "increase duration by 15 minutes for every two days there are approximately 70 to 75 percent successful voids." Note that children with developmental disorders often thrive on scheduling, but this is often based on routine activities rather than timed. If your child is used to picture cards indicating the order of events rather than a timed schedule, you can more easily adjust the amount of time between events without confusing them.

Ask a Parent

How do you handle potty training accidents?

"He won't pee in the potty at day care, only home. But I'm not backtracking just because they can't get him to pee. I'll bring him to work with me instead." —SABRINA

"I gave control to her: 'If you have to go pee pee, the potty is right over there. When you feel the pee pee about to come out, hold it and run to the potty and say, 'Pee pee coming.'" —EDITH

"It took a month of potty training for my daughter to tell me when she needed to go; before that I set a timer for every 45 minutes. She still occasionally has accidents but is going pretty well." —MASHA

THIRTEEN

Seeking Help

WHERE TO FIND MORE HELP

For starters, let's all be a little humble. Sometimes we need help. Whether it's help with kids, cleaning, or potty training, we've all been there. There is no shame in seeking additional help.

You may want to seek outside help if you find yourself in one or more of these situations:

- No progress forward or backward, just stuck in the same spot
- Sudden backsliding or accidents
- Noticeable changes in voiding or bowel habits
- Not sure what to do next
- Feeling like you've tried everything and nothing is working
- Feeling like you know the options, but are not sure which to take
- Had success with older children, but younger child is a different scenario
- Special-needs child
- If it takes more than one week for noticeable daytime progress or more than one month for noticeable nap or nighttime progress

For generations, people have taught pottying without doing it all alone. They grew up watching multiple other siblings, or nieces and nephews, being potty trained. They had aunts and grandmas and siblings to help. Asking for help is basically like job training. When I worked in "corporate America" my company paid to train me not only within my company but through a university as well. Think of potty training help like that. Your family is paying for you to learn how to do your job more efficiently, to the benefit of the whole family.

HOW TO FIND OUTSIDE SUPPORT WITH POTTY TRAINING:

- Online, from mommy blogs to support groups (see the Resources section on page 153 at the back)
- Friends with already potty trained kids
- Friends in the trenches of potty training with you (again, see the Resources section on page 153 at the back)
- Resources (like books, potty training video courses, articles, and others)
- Consultations with medical professionals. There are many reasons to seek medical advice, like poo or pee colors are outside of the normal range (see Chapter 6: Pooping and Peeing, page 80), abnormally frequent urinating, chronic constipation, "leaking" poop accidents, referral by a pediatrician for specific problem, and bedwetting (see Chapter 12: Accidents and Backsliding, page 134).
- Consultation with The Potty School. People come to me when they don't know where to start; they've started, but don't know what to do next; they've been failed by the support system they have for their child (whether it be family, support services, or others); they want a system catered specifically to their family and child; or they are behavioral therapists, psychologist, or doctors themselves.

Starting Over?

There is a time and place for scrapping it all and starting afresh. Typically, that time and place are not while potty training at home. If you tweak a method or type of motivation, you don't need to start over. However, if you haven't had success and are going to begin with a completely new method, you may want to start over again. It's fine to take a few diapering days in between to restart the process. Just keep your child up-to-date on what's going on, and be willing to take them to the potty while wearing their diaper as well. Most of the time, starting over is unnecessary and can be counterproductive, unless *you* really need the break.

Last-Ditch Effort

I give credence to the advice of parents, professionals, doctors, and traditions, even if not medically based . . . if it works. Before you throw in the towel, why not take a little advice from Grandma's generation and try out some "pee or poo drops." It's just sugar water in a dropper, taken like "medicine" to help your child go potty, get the pee in the toilet, not wet the bed, and so on. If that doesn't work, I look forward to talking with you soon!

FAQ

I've tried everything but nothing's worked. Now what?

You could keep online searching. You could complain or vent. You could seek wisdom. I have a friend who is studying to be a midwife. She chose her profession because as a young wife in her 20s she lost her husband in a fatal car accident. After that, she switched careers and decided to choose a profession where she gets to celebrate each and every life. What pregnant woman wouldn't want a support person like her to rely on, ask questions of, glean wisdom from, or be encouraged by about her baby's life? I'd like to think I'm a fraction of who my friend is to her clients. I am baffled by the amount of information I know about potty training. When I sit down and think about it, it makes me laugh. Who would have ever thought? I can get you to your next step. Just ask for help.

Should I talk to a doctor or a potty training professional?

I always recommend routine and as-needed visits with your child's pediatrician. If your pediatrician has no health concerns about your child, the frequent refrain is often to just wait a bit longer if potty training doesn't take within a few days. I have often consulted with parents who have been told to wait just a little longer. But this can add up to one, two, three, or even four years of waiting until their child is ready. Typically speaking, your doctor doesn't really care when your child is potty trained, as long as they are not having medical issues (such as UTIs or chronic constipation). There's no real motivation to push for potty training until it becomes a social stigma (around the time of entering preschool).

If your pediatrician specifically says that your child needs to go see a pediatric gastroenterologist, pediatric urologist, or any other specialist, you should start calling to book an appointment now. Because they are such niche specialties, the wait for a first visit can often be several weeks, and in some cases well over a month. In many cases a child can be potty trained while waiting on a specialist appointment.

If your child is deemed healthy by their pediatrician, there probably isn't further need of medical advice for potty training. As a potty training professional, I spend my days specifically learning the ins and outs of potty training in much more detail than a typical pediatrician would have need for. A potty training professional is well worth your time to give you a heads-up on best practices, fast-track your next steps, alleviate concerns, and expedite the pottying independence process.

Ask a Parent

When did you realize you needed help with potty training, and how did you find it?

"I Googled 'potty training professional' and found The Potty School." —JAMIE

"I'm a doctor and my wife is a nurse. We both helped potty train our daughter. We hit a dead end after a visit to her pediatrician when we talked about all the medical options to help her with poop training. I just needed someone to walk through the medical suggestions from a practical standpoint as to what's most likely to work before medical intervention is necessary. Within a month we went from daily accidents to my daughter going back to school with her twin brother (she had to leave school because of all the accidents). We were paying for her private preschool, even though she wasn't attending . . . and also paying for a nanny at home for her as well. From a one-hour phone consultation everything changed." —SHAWN

"We've given him MiraLAX over the spring/summer, but never really saw any 'results,' just a more peanut-buttery-textured poop, in his pants . . . definitely going to call a pediatric GI [gastroenterologist] tomorrow. His regular pediatrician suggested it awhile back if things didn't improve over the summer." —DENISE

"I called my mom crying because of being so frustrated about how potty training was going. We were getting nowhere fast. My mom actually looked up potty training help in Orange County and found The Potty School. She booked the consultation for me. After that consult, my son never peed on the ground or in his pants again!" —WANDA

Is seeking the help of a potty training professional actually going to help?

Yes and no. If you are willing to be honest about what has and hasn't worked, accept suggestions, and try something new, then it will be of the utmost help to you. If you think you have already read everything and know all the tricks, then the answer is probably no.

Is hiring a potty training consultant actually worth the money?

The answer is hands-down, "Yes!" Most families in the United States spend anywhere from $50 to $100 a month on diapers. A single consultation often cuts down on overall diapering needs by one to two months. That equals a cost savings of $100 to $200.

In-home training is a different ball game. It's not a dollar-for-dollar exchange. It's an investment in your child and in your family. Many who prefer in-home help are parents who have tried potty training without success, parents who want to get it done the right way the first time, or parents of a child with special needs. It's not a cop-out. It's an opportunity to have an expert co-parent along with you.

Conclusion
You Did It!

If I could hop off of this page and give you the kind of encouragement that makes you feel the most loved, I would! Don't you just want to celebrate? We'd LOVE to know when you've gotten to your Never Diaper: the next diaper that your child *would have used, but isn't going to* because they're done.

As a parent, I know you're busy, but I'd still love to celebrate with you! Go grab that last diaper that you're never going to use and do this:

- Grab a Sharpie
- Write #NeverDiaper #ThePottySchool
- Post on social media so we can find it and give you a digital high five!

Whoohoo! You're now saving anywhere from $50 to $100 per month on diapers! Not to mention the huge props my future great-grandchildren are giving you on reducing your family's eco-footprint

If you had someone else involved in the process, please take a quick second to thank them. Potty training is often a thankless job. Personally, I know I always appreciate getting updates from clients at info@thepotty school.com. If you have a quick second to drop me a line, I'd love to hear how I helped along the journey.

Congrats to you and your little one! I'm so honored to be a part of your pottying journey, and I would love to help a friend or family member of yours as well!

Appendix A

Potty Tracker

TIME OF DAY	PEE		
	Where did it go?		
	IN POTTY	PART IN POTTY	ALL IN CLOTHES/ ON FLOOR

POO

MOTIVATOR GIVEN?

Where did it go?

Yes/No

IN POTTY	PART IN POTTY	ALL IN CLOTHES/ ON FLOOR	

Training Checklist

☐ You, the parent, are ready
☐ You have a potty training plan
☐ Your house is prepared
☐ Your child is ready (you know what's reasonable to expect of them for their developmental stage/age)
☐ Your caregivers are prepared (preschool, day care, child care, etc.)
☐ Your child has nighttime poop control
☐ Your child has daytime poop control
☐ Your child has daytime pee control (wears undies during the day)
☐ You know that accidents and backsliding are possible
☐ Your child has nighttime pee control (wears undies at night)

Consider each checked box a victory along the journey to success in pottying.

Resources

The Potty School WWW.THEPOTTYSCHOOL.COM

Have a kiddo in diapers? Get potty training help anytime. We'll help you figure out the best next steps for your family. We offer free articles, DIY resources, personalized consultations (phone, video chat, and in-home) and help for all levels of support, from diapers to flush.

THE COMPLETE GUIDE TO POTTY TRAINING YOUR TODDLER ONLINE RESOURCES:

The Potty School's online resources complement this book and your potty training journey. They include visual guides, checklists, logs, and other tools and encouragement!
WWW.THEPOTTYSCHOOL.COM/POTTY-TRAINING-RESOURCES

THE POTTY SCHOOL'S POTTY TRAINING SUPPORT GROUP (AGES 18+ MONTHS):

Come join thousands of other parents on this journey with you! It's a place to be encouraged, lend a listening ear, and gain insight into tips and tricks others are using.
WWW.FACEBOOK.COM/GROUPS/POTTYTRAININGSUPPORTGROUP

Safety

WWW.AAP.ORG/EN-US/ADVOCACY-AND-POLICY/AAP-HEALTH-INITIATIVES/PRACTICING-SAFETY /PAGES/TOILET-TRAINING.ASPX

2-1-1 WWW.211.ORG

If you're in need of diapering or potty training supplies along the journey, 2-1-1 is a resource that provides basic necessities across the United States and parts of Canada. Help is offered for emergencies and disasters, food, crisis, health, housing and utilities, human trafficking, jobs and employment, reentry, and veterans.

Developmental Delays WWW.KENNEDYKRIEGER.ORG

Kennedy Krieger is dedicated to improving the lives of children and young adults with pediatric developmental disabilities and disorders of the brain, spinal cord, and musculoskeletal system, through patient care, special education, research, and professional training.

Visual Guide to Using the Bathroom

Available for free download at WWW.THEPOTTYSCHOOL.COM/VISUAL-GUIDE.

Diaper Bank WWW.NATIONALDIAPERBANKNETWORK.ORG/MEMBERS

Have some leftover diapers your child outgrew? Your local diaper bank can use them. Opened packages are fine, too. To find a drop-off point near you, email info@diaperbanknetwork.org.

Eating WWW.THEPOTTYSCHOOL.COM/VEGGIES

Have a picky eater? Poor nutrition can lead to constipation, diarrhea, pain while stooling, and even a fear of using the potty altogether. Jennifer Zils can guide your family to better eating habits with this resource.

Elimination Communication Resources
WWW.FACEBOOK.COM/GROUPS/ELIMINATIONCOMMUNICATIONSUPPORTGROUP

Join The Potty School's Elimination Communication Support Group
(ages 0–18 months). It's a place to be encouraged, lend a listening ear, and
gain insight into tips and tricks others are using.

Love WWW.5LOVELANGUAGES.COM

Love is not outdated. Learning how to connect with your child in the way
they feel most appreciated and encouraged will be hugely helpful along
your potty training and parenting journey.

Safe Families for Children WWW.SAFE-FAMILIES.ORG

Our family has hosted several children in our home through this
organization, and we have been grateful for each and every child's
days spent with us.

Safe Families for Children is a movement fueled by compassion to
keep children safe and families intact. Through host families, family
friends, and family coaches, the network temporarily hosts children and
provides a network of support to families in crisis while they get back on
their feet.

Refer a Family in Need:
WWW.SAFE-FAMILIES.ORG/GET-HELP/REFER-A-FAMILY-IN-NEED

Request a Host Family:
WWW.SAFE-FAMILIES.ORG/GET-HELP/REQUEST-A-HOST-FAMILY

Sleep WWW.THEPOTTYSCHOOL.COM/BABYSLEEPSITE

Baby not sleeping? Get sleep help around the clock with free e-books, blogs, DIY resources, and one-on-one personalized sleep consultations. The Baby Sleep Site has practical, nonjudgmental advice for every type of family!

The ChildHelp National Child Abuse Hotline
WWW.CHILDHELP.ORG/HOTLINE/

1-800-4-A-CHILD or 1-800-422-4453

PEE
▬▬▬▬

Daytime Continence

Children's Hospital of Orange County: Provides free videos, audio, and paid medical services, including behavioral therapy, pelvic floor rehabilitation, medication, surgery, and dietary modifications. WWW.THEPOTTYSCHOOL.COM/CHOC

University of California, Los Angeles: Jennifer Singer, MD, who wrote the introduction to this book, is a pediatric urologist at UCLA. I can personally recommend her help if you are in need of a pediatric urologist. She is both a practicing physician and a clinical professor. WWW.UCLAHEALTH.ORG/JENNIFER-SINGER

Yale: Patient treatments include urotherapy, transcutaneous electrical nerve stimulation (TENS), biofeedback, medications, counseling, clinical trials, and surgery. WWW.THEPOTTYSCHOOL.COM/YALE

Bedwetting WWW.EN.WIKIPEDIA.ORG/WIKI/NOCTURNAL_ENURESIS

Use the above resource for basic facts about bedwetting. You can also consult the article "Definition & Facts for Bladder Control Problem & Bedwetting in Children" by the U.S. Department of Health and Human Services.
WWW.NIDDK.NIH.GOV/HEALTH-INFORMATION/UROLOGIC-DISEASES/BLADDER-CONTROL
-PROBLEMS-BEDWETTING-CHILDREN/DEFINITION-FACTS

POOP

WWW.THEPOTTYSCHOOL.COM/DR-POO

Dr. Poo is a comprehensive but easily readable e-book about how and why we poop by Dr. William Sears.

References

Bayne, Aaron P., and Steven J. Skoog. "Nocturnal Enuresis: An Approach to Assessment and Treatment." *Pediatrics in Review* 35, no. 8 (August 2014): 327–34. doi:10.1542/pir.35-8-327.

Borowitz, Stephen M. "Pediatric Constipation Differential Diagnoses." Medscape. Accessed February 14, 2018. https://emedicine.staging .medscape.com/article/928185-differential.

Chengappa, Karishma. "Toilet Training Children with Autism Spectrum Disorders." March 26, 2018. https://www.kennedykrieger.org/sites /default/files/star_training/card-toilet-training-chengappa.pdf.

Cincinnati Children's Hospital. "Cognitive Development." Accessed February 12, 2018. https://www.cincinnatichildrens.org/health /c/cognitive.

Davis, Susan. "Potty Training: Seven Surprising Facts." WebMD. Accessed January 3, 2018. https://www.webmd.com/parenting /features/potty-training-seven-surprising-facts#1.

Goode, Erica. "Two Experts Do Battle over Potty Training." *New York Times*, January 12, 1999. http://www.nytimes.com/1999/01/12/us /two-experts-do-battle-over-potty-training.html.

Graham, Katherine M., and Jay B. Levy. "Enuresis." *Pediatrics in Review* 30, no. 5 (May 2009). http://pedsinreview.aappublications .org/content/30/5/165.

Hodges, Steve J., and Evelyn Y. Anthony. "Occult Megarectum: A Commonly Unrecognized Cause of Enuresis." *Urology* 79, no. 2 (February 2012): 421–24. doi:10.1016/j.urology.2011.10.015.

"Important Milestones: Your Child By Five Years." Centers for Disease Control and Prevention. October 25, 2017. Accessed May 5, 2018. https://www.cdc.gov/ncbddd/actearly/milestones/milestones-5yr.html.

Kiddoo, Darcie A. "Toilet Training Children: When to Start and How to Train." *Canadian Medical Association Journal* 184, no. 5 (March 2012): 511. doi:10.1503.cmaj.110830.

National Institute of Diabetes and Digestive and Kidney Diseases. "Definition & Facts for Bladder Control Problems & Bedwetting in Children." September 2017. https://www.niddk.nih.gov/health-information/urologic-diseases/bladder-control-problems-bedwetting-children/definition-facts.

Nguyen, Thai. "Success Starts with Self-Mastery: 7 Effective Strategies." Accessed December 30, 2017. https://www.skipprichard.com/success-starts-with-self-mastery-7-effective-strategies/.

Olson, Andrea. *Go Diaper Free: A Simple Handbook for Elimination Communication.* Asheville, NC: The Tiny World Company, 2013.

Pampers. "7 Signs Your Child Is Ready to Potty Train." January 31, 2018. https://www.pampers.com/en-us/toddler/potty-training/article/7-signs-your-child-is-ready-to-potty-train.

Pérez, M. Minguez, and A. Benages Martínez. "The Bristol Scale: A Useful System to Access Stool Form" *Spanish Journal of Digestive Diseases* 101, no. 5 (May 2009). Accessed February 14, 2018. http://scielo.isciii.es/scielo.php?script=sci_arttext&pid=S1130-01082009000500001&lng=en&nrm=iso&tlng=en.

Polland, Barbara K. *No Directions on the Package: A Practical Guide for Parents.* Berkeley, CA: Celestial Arts, 2000.

Schmitt, Barton D. "Toilet Training: Getting It Right the First Time." *Contemporary Pediatrics.* March 2004. Accessed February 14, 2018. http://contemporarypediatrics.modernmedicine.com/contemporary-pediatrics/news/clinical/pediatrics/toilet-training-getting-it-right-first-time.

Stadtler, Ann C., Peter A. Gorski, and T. Berry Brazelton. "Toilet Training Methods, Clinical Interventions, and Recommendations." *Pediatrics* 103, supplement 3 (June 1999). http://pediatrics.aap publications.org/content/103/Supplement_3/1359.

"Stools—Foul Smelling." United States National Library of Medicine. Accessed February 14, 2018. https://medlineplus.gov/ency /article/003132.htm.

Teyber, Edward, and Faith Teyber. *Interpersonal Process in Therapy: An Integrative Model*. Boston: Cengage Learning, 2010.

Thaman, Lauren A., and Lawrence F. Eichenfield. "Diapering Habits: A Global Perspective." *Pediatric Dermatology* 31, supplement 1 (2014): 15–18. doi:10.1111/pde.12468.

"Toilet Training." American Academy of Pediatrics. Accessed February 14, 2018. https://www.aap.org/en-us/advocacy-and-policy/ aap-health-initiatives/practicing-safety/Pages/Toilet-Training.aspx.

"Urine – Abnormal Color." United States National Library of Medicine. Accessed February 14, 2018. https://medlineplus.gov/ency/article /003139.htm.

USDA Food Composition Database. United States Department of Agriculture Agricultural Research Service. Accessed February 14, 2018. https://ndb.nal.usda.gov/.

Yeung, C.K., and Jennifer D.Y. Sihoe. "Non-Neuropathic Dysfunction of the Lower Urinary Tract in Children." Edited by W. Scott McDougal. In *Campbell-Walsh Urology 10th Edition Review*. Philadelphia, PA: Saunders, 2011.

Zoppi, G., M. Cinquetti, A. Luciano, A. Benini, A. Muner, and Minelli E. Bertazzoni. "The Intestinal Ecosystem in Chronic Functional Constipation." *Acta Paediatrica* 87, no. 8 (August 1998): 836–41. doi:10.1111/j.1651-2227.1998.tb01547.x.

Index

About the Author

MICHELLE D. SWANEY is the CEO of The Potty School, a potty training consultant, and a sought-after event speaker. She helps parents move toward the next step on their family's pottying journey . . . from diapers to flush.

Michelle is passionate about helping parents to embrace their "pottying personality" in order to potty train with a style and method that is most effective, and enjoyable, for their family and specific child. That leads to pottying independence, while making the journey one based on building a bond and connection with their child.

Michelle doesn't do her job because she *loves* pee and poo, but she does it because she *loves* being able to help parents learn to communicate with their children from a young age and *loves* to reduce children's dependence upon diapers. Curtailing diaper use has saved her clients an average of $50 to $100 per month, while simultaneously reducing their eco-footprint—two great reasons to smile!

Michelle is your go-to gal when it comes to anything pottying. She is the wife of Matt, and mother of Timothy, Poema, and Sierra. She resides in Orange County, California.

CPSIA information can be obtained
at www.ICGtesting.com
Printed in the USA
BVHW06s0314140618
518892BV00002B/2/P